Nursing Care Planning Guides
Set 3
Second Edition

Nursing Care Planning Guides
Set 3
Second Edition

Margo Creighton Neal, RN, MN
VICE PRESIDENT, WILLIAMS & WILKINS

Patricia Feltz Cohen, RN, MA, EdM
CONSULTANT, HUNTINGTON BEACH, CA

Joan Reighley, RN, MN
PSYCHOTHERAPIST, PRIVATE PRACTICE, LOS ANGELES, CA
Certified, specialist; Division of Psychiatric and Mental Health Nursing,
American Nurses' Association

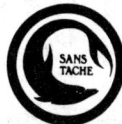

WILLIAMS & WILKINS
Baltimore • London • Los Angeles • Sydney

Contributing Author   Elizabeth M. DeSantis, RN, MS

Copyright © 1983—Margo Creighton Neal
Copyright © 1985—Williams & Wilkins
428 East Preston Street, Baltimore, Maryland 21202 U.S.A.

Printed in the United States of America

Library of Congress Cataloging in Publication Data

Main entry under title:
Nursing care planning guides, set 3, 2nd Ed.

    1. Nursing—Handbooks, manuals, etc. 2. Nursing—Planning—Handbooks, manuals, etc. I. Neal, Margo Creighton, 1935–
II. Cohen, Patricia Feltz, 1932–   . III. Reighley, Joan, 1936–   . IV. Title.
[DNLM: 1. Patient care planning—Handbooks. 2. Nursing care—Handbooks. WY 100 N342n 1980]
RT51.N3715   1982   610.73   82-14316
ISBN 0-683-09521-8

    86 87 88 89   10 9 8 7 6 5 4

Set No. 3
TABLE OF CONTENTS

PREFACE

The nursing care plan continues to provide the most reliable source of information regarding the assessment and planning of nursing care in hospitals and health care agencies. The Joint Commission on Accreditation of Hospitals has mandated nursing care plans for a long time; in recent years they have come to look at them more critically and rigorously during the accreditation process. More and more nurses practicing today were taught the nursing process and the resulting nursing care plan in their generic RN programs. Many others learned the process in continuing education courses; yet the actual writing and implementation of nursing care plans remain somewhat elusive, time-consuming, and inconsistent.

Thousands of nurses have found the NURSECO *Nursing Care Planning Guides* to be invaluable aids in streamlining this cumbersome process. This 2nd Edition of Set 3 updates and expands on 50 of them. The hand-picked selection of Medical-Surgical Conditions, Maternal-Child Health Situations, Psychiatric and Mental Health Conditions, plus selected Supplementary Information Guides, will be a useful addition to nursing care units. It will provide easy to read, quickly accessed, pertinent information in a form that adapts itself readily to the needs of the nursing process and nursing care plan.

Each Guide, except for those in the Supplementary Information, contains these components: *General Considerations* to refresh the nurse's knowledge base about the specific disease/condition and to help in patient assessment; *Specific Considerations,* containing nursing diagnoses categories, potential patient outcomes, and possible nursing actions; *Discharge Planning and Teaching Objectives/Outcomes* that are outlines for patient education, convalescence, and health maintenance; and *Recommended References,* an up-to-date list of articles on nursing care of patients with this particular disease/condition. Each Supplementary Information Guide enhances the other Guides.

In this edition, we attempted to avoid stereotyping the nurse as "she" and the patient as "he" by using "s/he" in lieu of she/he. However, the English language has not yet produced a combination form for masculine and feminine pronouns, thus you will note some referral to the patient in the masculine form only.

This 2nd Edition of Set 3 is cross referenced to the four other fine collections of Nursing Care Planning Guides in this series. They are a valuable addition to any nursing unit.

Margo C. Neal
Patricia F. Cohen
Joan Reighley

INTRODUCTION

Use these Nursing Care Planning Guides to produce a workable nursing care plan. It requires a little practice, but once the technique is mastered you will not only find them invaluable, you will also enjoy the process.

To use these Guides, select a Nursing Care Planning Guide for a condition normally encountered in your practice, e.g., #3:09, "The Patient with Low Back Pain," and scan its contents. The *General Considerations* will help you do the patient assessment. Use the *Specific Considerations* to devise accurate nursing diagnoses. If the patient has an actual or potential problem in one of them (e.g., "Rest/Relaxation"), make the specific nursing diagnosis ("Impaired Physical Mobility"). Next, specify an expected outcome for the nursing diagnosis; choose one of those suggested, or develop a new one. Then select the nursing actions that will help the patient achieve the desired outcomes; again, choose from those in the Guide or specify your own. The *Discharge Planning and Teaching Objectives/Outcomes* list potential education and discharge goals; they will help you develop a strategy that can be implemented well in advance of the day the patient goes home.

Use the Supplementary Information Guides to enhance the above (e.g., NCPGs #3:41, "Back Care: General Principles," and #3:42, "Back Exercises"). Review the cross reference to the other four sets of *Nursing Care Planning Guides* as indicated and needed.

With these quick reference, up-to-date Guides, producing a comprehensive, usable care plan in a minimum amount of time now becomes possible.

These *Nursing Care Planning Guides* are meant to *guide* you in writing nursing care plans that are individualized to a specific patient. Therefore, select and use those parts that you judge appropriate to your patient. Add to them as the patient's condition and responses to your nursing actions dictate. Use these Guides to enhance your own professional judgment.

The Patient Having an Abortion

Definition: Abortion is the termination of a pregnancy before the fetus is theoretically viable.

LONG TERM GOAL: The patient will return to her usual roles in home/job/community, free of preventable complications and will express a degree of confidence in the decision made about terminating her pregnancy.

General Considerations:

— Abortions (AB) may be **classified** or labeled as:
  - *Spontaneous* (occurring naturally without interference): a spontaneous AB may be *threatened* (not yet occurred), *incomplete* (some of the products of pregnancy are retained in utero), *complete, inevitable,* or *missed* (the fetus dies in utero, but is not expelled). Approximately one of every 10 pregnancies ends in spontaneous abortion.
  - *Habitual*: the woman has three or more spontaneous abortions.
  - *Therapeutic* (legal or induced AB): termination of a pregnancy by a physician in a medical facility.
  - *Criminal*: the illegal termination of a pregnancy by the patient or others.

— The term "abortion" is widely used to designate interruption of a pregnancy before the fetus is viable (± 28 weeks gestation; legal periods of viability vary from state to state in the US); expulsion of the fetus after this time is called "premature birth."

— The term "miscarriage" is widely used in lay language to refer to spontaneous abortion; today, "abortion" in lay language may refer to legal, illegal, criminal, or artificial abortion.

— Abortion **techniques** include:
  1) *D&C*: A surgical procedure in which the cervix is dilated and the wall of the uterus scraped to empty the contents. It is usually done up to 12 weeks gestation (see NCPG #3:02).
  2) *Suction aspiration or vacuum curretage*: the cervix is dilated and a suction catheter is passed into the uterus in order to aspirate the conceptual material. Used up to 12 weeks gestation only, often in out-patient settings.
  3) *Hysterotomy*: like a mini "C-section," it is usually done between 12–24 weeks gestation when the fetus is too large to ensure a safe passage through the softened cervix, thus eliminating techniques 1) and 2) above. This technique is being replaced with 4) and 5) below with increasing frequency.

4) *Hypertonic saline*: removal of amniotic fluid and replacement of it with a 20% hypertonic saline solution, via needle through the abdominal wall, mid-line below the umbilicus. Within 12–16 hours the fetus dies, labor begins, and the products of conception are expelled. Used from 12–24 weeks gestation.

5) *Prostaglandins*: administration of extra amniotic prostaglandin into the space between the amniotic sac and the uterine wall, usually via a Foley catheter through the cervix and into the uterus. As with 4) above, the procedure usually results in delivery of the fetus within 16–20 hours; may be used during the first 26 weeks of pregnancy.

— Most legal abortions are done by the 12th week of gestation (first trimester) when the risks of complications are minimal.

— The three **main dangers of illegal abortion** are rupture of the cervix, hemorrhage, and infection. The actual number of illegal abortions performed each year is not known. Legal abortions have increased from 615,831 in 1973 to 1,157,776 in 1978 (US Dept. of Health & Human Services).

— In January 1973, the US Supreme Court ruled that a pregnancy may be terminated under the following conditions:

1) during the first trimester, the abortion or decision is left to the woman and her doctor;

2) during the second trimester, the state may not prohibit abortion but may *regulate* it in the interest of protecting the woman's health;

3) during the third trimester, the state may choose to protect the life of the fetus by prohibiting abortion except when necessary to preserve the life or health of the woman;

4) the religious beliefs of the woman are always respected.

— What does the landmark US Supreme Court ruling mean for you, the nurse? Many health team members have strong, negative, and/or ambivalent feelings about abortion. The most important thing for you to identify is your own feelings and beliefs regarding abortion. If you are opposed to induced abortion, feelings will invariably be communicated to the patient via words, body language, attitudes, etc. If you feel you cannot participate in any aspect of an abortion procedure and/or subsequent care of the patient, it is your responsibility to inform the nursing office so that you will not be placed in a conflicting, uncomfortable situation.

Specific Considerations, Potential Patient Outcomes, and Nursing Actions:

1) Pre-abortion Assessment (Anxiety, Lack of Knowledge, Signs of Spontaneous AB)

The patient will experience no more than a moderate amount of anxiety; the patient will receive supportive, non-judgmental nursing care; the patient will receive as much information as she wants and needs to know re: the selected abortion technique:
— observe pt. for signs of anxiety (e.g., nervousness, restlessness, asking same questions over & over, rapid pulse, constant talking); ask her to tell you what she is feeling just now; listen to & accept what she says; what is the focus or theme of what she is saying? acknowledge her feelings & share with her that other pts. in a similar situation feel as she does;
— if a therapeutic AB, ask her if she wishes to share the rationale for her decision with you; accept & support her in what she says;
— ask her to tell you what she knows about the selected AB technique; correct any misinformation & ask her what else she would like to know; provide as much information as she wishes, including post-abortion expectations; do not give all this information before assessment (sometimes providing more than the pt. wants to know will only increase anxiety);
— ask her what you could do for her to increase her comfort; provide it, if at all possible, or work out an acceptable substitute;
— if pt. is having a spontaneous abortion, assess abdominal cramps, bleeding (including pad count), signs of shock, & report to MD; have pt. use bedpan in lieu of bathroom & send vaginal discharge to lab for examination of tissue; provide bed rest & prevent straining on defecation; keep pt. NPO unless otherwise ordered (may need a D&C).

2) Post-abortion Prevention of Complications

The patient will experience a smooth post-abortion course, free of preventable complications (e.g., shock, profuse bleeding, infection):
— observe pt. post-abortion for bleeding, changes in vital signs, abdominal cramps, signs of shock; report to MD PRN;
— if patient had a D&C, review NCPG #3:02;
— observe for signs of complications specific to a hypertonic saline abortion:

- *hypernatremia* (as a result of injection of the saline solution into the blood stream): common manifestations, which may follow the injection within one minute, are dry mouth, flushed face, tinnitis, heat sensation, tachycardia, or severe headache. Should this occur, the saline injection is stopped & an IV of D_5W started; after an uncomplicated saline infusion, pts. are instructed to drink at least 2 liters of H_2O over the next 12 hours to prevent hypernatremia;
- *peritoneal spill* (some of the saline solution spills into the peritoneal cavity, usually when the needle is being removed or from a leak at the amniocentesis site): severe abdominal pain, tachycardia, thirst; usually treated with an IV of D_5W & water by mouth;
- *bladder infection* (resulting from misplacement of needle into bladder): manifested by backache, burning, & urgency 10–15 seconds after injection is started; usually treated with immediate irrigation of bladder with normal saline;
— after fetus is expelled, clamp & cut cord, remove fetus from bedside & send to lab; if pt. asks to see it, show it to her; if she asks sex of fetus, & it is discernible, tell her; placenta should be expelled within 2 hours; if not, notify MD (a D&C may be required);
— after placenta is expelled, send it to lab; massage & palpate fundus Q15 minutes PRN, then Q4H PRN; give perineal care Q4H & PRN.

3) Psycho-social Adjustment

The patient will grieve adaptively over the loss of her pregnancy and will be supported in this by the nursing staff:
— know that the woman's response to her loss will depend to a great measure on whether or not the pregnancy was desired: she may view the abortion as a great loss or a great relief; in either case, the pt. will experience some degree of depression & may be angry; this anger may be projected onto you; when this happens, be aware that it is not meant for you personally; acknowledge the pt.'s anger, but do not react to it;
— provide empathic listening & acceptance of what the pt. says; acknowledge her feelings & encourage her to continue ("You seem upset. Can you tell me more about it?"); share with her that other women in a similar situation often feel as she does;
— review NCPG #1:31, "Responses to Loss: The Grief & Mourning Process."

Discharge Planning and Teaching Objectives/Outcomes

1) (Patient/Family/Significant Other) Can demonstrate proper perineal care and knows importance of it as a preventative to infection.
2) Verbalizes feelings regarding loss of fetus to staff and/or family/significant other.
3) Knows when she can resume use of tampons, douching, coitus (usually 4-6 weeks), and knows that it is possible to become pregnant again within 2-3 weeks.
4) Has an appointment with doctor/clinic for follow-up care.
5) Knows that vaginal bleeding may continue for a week, and to call doctor if it lasts longer than 10 days; knows to call if there is bright red bleeding at any time; knows signs of infection (temperature, severe uterine cramping, foul odor, discharge) and to call doctor PRN.
6) Has been offered and/or given contraceptive counseling.
7) If patient is discharged after a saline infusion, has received instructions to either (a) return to medical facility when abortion is imminent, or (b) to monitor abortion at home and report to doctor or clinic.

Recommended References

"Abortion Availability in the United States," by S. Seims. *Family Planning Perspective*, March/April 1980:88, 93-101.

"Abortion: Legal, Medical, and Social Perspectives," by J. Widdicombe et al. *Family Community Health*, November 1979:17-28.

"Birth Control: Permanent Methods & Temporary Methods." *NCP Guides #5:38, 39*, Nurseco, 1981.

"Competing Ethical Claims in Abortion," by A.J. Davis. *American Journal of Nursing*, July 1980:1359.

"Helping Staff Nurses Care for Women Seeking Saline Abortions," by M. Olson. *JOGN Nursing*, May/June 1980:170-174.

"Minor Consent in Birth-Control and Abortion," by D. Trandel-Karencheck et al. *Nurse Practitioner*, March/April 1980:47-54.

"The Patient Having a D&C." *NCP Guide #3:02*, 2nd Ed., Nurseco, 1983.

"Repeat Abortions: Blaming the Victim," by B. Howe et al. *The American Journal of Public Health*, July 1979:1242-1246.

"Responses to Loss: The Grief and Mourning Process." *NCP Guide #1:31*, 2nd Ed., Nurseco, 1980.

The Patient with a D&C (Dilatation and Curretage)

Definition: A D&C (dilatation and curretage) is a surgical procedure in which the cervix is dilated and the inner wall of the uterus is scraped.

LONG TERM GOAL: The patient will return to her usual roles in home/job/community, free of any preventable complications.

General Considerations:
— A D&C may be done for any of several reasons, including:
  - to obtain endometrial or endocervical tissue for cytology examination;
  - to control abnormal bleeding;
  - to terminate a pregnancy; or
  - to serve as a therapeutic measure in incomplete abortion.
— **Nursing responsibilities** include knowing the reason for the D&C, assessing the patient's knowledge and feelings regarding the procedure, providing effective post-op care, and health teaching the patient prior to discharge.

Specific Considerations, Potential Patient Outcomes, and Nursing Actions:

1) Pre-op Anxiety and Knowledge of Procedure

The patient will experience no more than a moderate amount of anxiety; the patient will receive as much information about the surgical procedure as she wants to know:
— ask pt. how she feels about having the D&C; provide empathic listening; provide support by asking her what it is like for her to be here just now;
— ask her what she thinks might make her feel better & provide it, if at all possible;
— assess pt.'s knowledge of D&C & desire to know more; health teach PRN; it is important to assess how much she *wants* to know, rather than just feeding information to her;
— know that a moderate amount of anxiety is exhibited by the pt. when she asks questions & accepts the information given, & when she has realistic expectations re: post-op pain, discomfort, & activity; when your pt. exhibits these behaviors, reassure her that these are usual & desirable;
— carry out procedures prescribed for this surgery by the hospital & pt.'s MD;
— review NCPG #2:44, "General Pre-op Care."

2) Post-op
   Care

The patient will experience an uneventful recovery, free of preventable complications (e.g., shock, infection):
— review NCPGs #2:41–43, "General Post-op Care;"
— observe for vaginal bleeding & report excessive amount to MD; provide sterile perineal pads & hold in place with sanitary belt; chart # of pads used & approximate amount of drainage (spotty, slight, moderate, or heavy); report excessive bleeding to MD;
— know that infection & hemorrhage are the main complications of a D&C; to aid prevention, change perineal pads frequently as the discharge makes a good medium for growth of bacteria; provide perineal care as long as there is discharge, or as MD orders;
— if pt. had D&C for an incomplete abortion, she may be having mild to severe cramps; share with her that these are usual & expected & will disappear; pelvic or low-back pain is also usual, & is often relieved with analgesics;
— measure I&O & record; assist pt. to bathroom for first post-op voiding & PRN thereafter; explain to pt. that she might feel faint after procedure, & it is best for her to call you to go to bathroom;
— provide bed rest with BR privileges for remainder of day;
— when pt. fully alert, ask her how she is feeling now; use your judgment to proceed as outlined in #1 above re: anxiety & feelings.

Discharge Planning and Teaching Objectives/Outcomes
1) (Patient/Family/Significant Other) Can verbalize an understanding of D&C and knows to contact doctor if vaginal bleeding continues more than seven days, or if develops a fever, and/or a foul-smelling vaginal discharge.
2) Has an appointment for follow-up care with doctor or clinic.
3) Is aware that the anesthetic can make her feel tired and to rest for next three days, walking or sitting as tolerated.
4) Verbalizes willingness to avoid heavy lifting, climbing stairs, or pushing heavy objects for three days.

Recommended References
"General Post-op Care: Parts A, B, C." *NCP Guides #2:41, 42, 43*, 2nd Ed., Nurseco, 1980.
"General Pre-op Care." *NCP Guide #2:44*, 2nd Ed., Nurseco, 1980.
"The Patient Having an Abortion." *NCP Guide #3:01*, 2nd Ed., Nurseco, 1983.

The Patient on Dialysis: Hemodialysis

Definition: Dialysis is the diffusion of solute molecules through a semipermeable membrane in an artificial kidney machine from the side of higher concentration to that of lower concentration.

LONG TERM GOAL: The patient will adhere to prescribed regimen to aid recovery from the acute renal failure and to return to usual roles; OR—the patient will adapt to the reality of long-term dialysis and will live within its accompanying limitations.

General Considerations:
— **Public Law 92-603 of July 1973** provides financial assistance under Medicaid to all persons covered by Social Security, or their dependents, who have end stage renal disease and who require dialysis (and/or kidney transplant). Approximately 60,000 persons in the US are being maintained on permanent dialysis.
— **Purpose:** to remove waste products from the blood and to maintain the life and well-being of the patient.
— **Principle indication** for dialysis is a high and rising serum K level; other indications include a severe fluid and/or electrolyte imbalance, severe pulmonary edema or congestive heart failure, chemical or drug toxicity. Dialysis may be done on an *emergency basis* (as in acute renal failure, drug or chemical toxicity), on a *long-term basis* (as in chronic renal failure), or on a *temporary basis* (while patient is waiting for a kidney transplant).
— **How does it work?** The artificial kidney contains a semipermeable membrane that separates the patient's blood from the dialyzing solutions (made by a delivery system). By the principles of diffusion and osmosis, molecules and ions of waste products pass from the area of higher concentration (the patient's blood) to the area of lower concentration (the dialyzing solution) until a degree of equilibrium between the two is achieved. Molecules may also pass from the dialyzing solution into the blood, thus the electrolyte content of the dialysate can be manipulated so as to meet the patient's needs based on blood chemistries and clinical evaluation.
— **Procedure:** access to the patient's circulation is achieved in one of two ways: (1) in *external shunting* (or cannulization), a silastic-teflon cannula is surgically inserted and fixed in an artery (usually the radial of the *nondominant arm* or posterior tibial); another cannula is fixed in a nearby vein. Arterial blood is shunted from the patient through the artificial kidney and returned to the patient via the venous cannula. After the dialysis is completed, the two cannulae are connected so that the flow of blood from artery to vein through the "shunt" is continuous. Types of external shunts: Scribner, Thomas, Busselmier. In (2) *internal shunting* (or

fistulization), a tiny opening is surgically created between an artery and a nearby vein; this enables the arterial blood to enter into and engorge the vein, which is then easily punctured at time of dialysis. Two needles are inserted, one to carry the blood to the artificial kidney, and one to return the blood to the patient. After the procedure, the needles are removed and reinserted for each treatment. No external device is used and problems of clotting and infection are minimized. Patency of the fistula is achieved by the rapid flow of blood through it. Types of internal shunts: fistula Cimino, bovine graft, Impra graft, Gortex, Bentley Biocarbon, and Hemasite fistula. Each method of shunting has advantages and disadvantages; the choice is affected by many variables. A properly cared for shunt can last many years.

— **Time involved** for hemodialysis is approximately three to five hours, depending on patient and type of machine used. It is usually done three times/week.

— **Nursing responsibilities** include monitoring the dialysis procedure to ensure a smooth operation, observing patient for signs of discomfort and potential complications, providing patient and family teaching and counseling, and by making clinical judgments to adjust prescription dialysis. Prepare yourself by becoming thoroughly acquainted with the set-up, nursing procedure manuals, complication and emergency procedures, and protocol for the unit; read all manufacturers' labels and instruction sheets; participate in health team conferences; use the inservice education department as a resource for additional information and assistance.

— **Caution:** hemodialysis patients require large amounts of blood transfusions, making them more susceptible to hepatitis B and hepatitis non-A and non-B. Exercise extreme caution when doing venipuncture, handling blood, or disposing of the patient's body excreta.

Specific Considerations, Potential Patient Outcomes, and Nursing Actions:

1) Preparation of Patient/ Comfort Measures

The patient will know what to expect in terms of length of treatment, discomfort, oral intake; the patient will be involved in planning own care to achieve physical and emotional comfort:
— assess pt.'s knowledge of procedure & give as much information as s/he requests & needs to know; speak in calm, reassuring tones;
— if initial access to pt.'s circulation is done, carefully explain this procedure to pt.;
— plan care with pt.; if s/he has been previously dialyzed, ask what you can do to make this treatment comfortable;
— provide frequent back rubs & massage pressure points PRN; pt. may be in bed or resting in chair, depending on condition;

— provide mouth care, personal hygiene, & diversionary activities PRN;
— inform pt. of signs of a smooth dialysis (e.g., good flow of blood, change in blood chemistries, etc.) so that s/he too may know progress;
— assess & chart pt.'s hydration status by analyzing weight, skin turgor, thirst, mucus membrane moisture, I&O, & edema; see NCPG #3:48, "Fluids" (It is very important to establish the pt.'s dry weight in order to determine inter- dialytic weight gain.).

2) Prevention of Compli- cations

The patient will receive an effective dialysis, free of preventable complications; if complications occur the patient will have them promptly detected and optimally managed:
— report to MD any signs & symptoms that are deviations from the acceptable range; know that common compli- cations, observations, & critical care include:

- *cerebral edema* due to too rapid removal of urea; observe for symptoms of disequilibrium (headache, N&V, mental confusion, hallucinations, convulsions, tremors); give analgesics, sedatives, or anticonvulsive drugs as ordered; protect pt. from injury during convulsions; dialysis may be slowed or discontinued if symptoms in- crease; Mannitol IV may be used during the first dialysis to prevent disequilibrium;

- *volume overload* with increased BP, related to IV blood, plasma expander, or saline given to support BP during dialysis, or rapid volume return to pt.'s system; observe for symptoms (engorged neck veins, tachycardia, in- creased BP & CVP, dyspnea, gallup rhythm, peripheral or cutaneous edema, rales); report to MD PRN; watch for shortness of breath (could indicate early pulmonary edema);

- *ultrafiltration* due to too rapid removal of fluid from the blood compartment (indicated by a low BP); at the be- ginning of dialysis, assess the pt. for optimal fluid loss & set UF pressures to ensure a gradual removal of fluid throughout the treatment; take BP, pulse QH, continuous weights PRN;

- *chest pain* may be caused by cardiac dysrhythmias, angina pectoris precipitated by electrolyte imbalance, low BP, air or blood embolus; note type, location, & precipitate of pain; encourage pt. to lie quietly in bed; have O_2 available; be familiar with hospital routine for cardiac arrest & emergency treatment for air embolus;

- *circulatory shock* (indicated by decreased BP, N&V, faintness): take BP PRN, medicate as ordered; follow unit protocol & be familiar with unit procedures for cardiac arrest;

- *clotting/bleeding*: monitor pt. for signs of bleeding, check equipment for signs of clotting, & monitor coagulation levels according to unit protocol; inform pt. that heparin requires about 4 hours postdialysis to metabolize & that s/he should watch for signs of shunt bleeding & avoid cuts, bumps during this time;
- *hemolysis*: record carefully predialysis machine disinfecting test, machine conductivity, & temperature in accordance with unit protocol & policy;
— monitor vital signs, blood flow, mental status at least QH & PRN.

3) Fluids and Electrolytes

The patient will be free of preventable fluid and electrolyte imbalance during dialysis:
— record very accurately all intake (IV, oral fluids), output (urine, vomitus, perspiration), & whether pt. has had his dialyzer prime bled;
— provide fluids strictly as ordered; amount will vary with each pt.; give only those permitted in diet;
— draw blood samples as ordered, know normal ranges, record results & report to MD;
— weigh pt. according to unit protocol with same clothing & using same scale;
— read NCPGs #3:48 & 49, "Fluids & Electrolytes."

4) Psycho-social Adjustment (to Dependency on Dialysis)

The patient will continue to deal adaptively with changes in body image and usual role functioning; the patient will accept and adapt to maintenance dialysis; the patient will be responsible for managing own care:
— read NCPG #3:14, "Chronic Renal Failure," Psychosocial Adjustment (consideration #4);
— observe pt.'s affect & mental status before dialysis begins; is s/he sad? happy? feeling helpless or hopeless? anxious? validate your observations with the pt. ("You seem down today; are you?") as a way of getting pt. to express feelings; provide empathic listening;
— be aware that dialysis pts. usually follow a pattern of (1) feeling increasingly better physically during first few weeks or months of dialysis; (2) then becoming discouraged & easily depressed; followed by (3) some degree of acceptance of medical condition & imposed limitations, evidenced by a lessening of negative feelings & planning for changes in life style; determine where your pt. is in this pattern & discuss it with both pt. & family; review NCPGs #1:20–33 on patient behaviors; maintain realistic time frame for pattern in each patient;
— prevent communication breakdown by setting up family, pt., & staff conferences with psychiatric clinical specialist, psychiatrist, social worker, or other mental health person;

— know that dialysis pts. usually have many conflicts re: being dependent on a machine & health team for life, & that these may be expressed by a variety of feelings & emotions; accept & acknowledge all verbalizations the pt. gives; tell pt. that these are usual & expected feelings for dialysis pts.; acceptance of pt.'s feelings by the nurse will often keep the pt. from acting them out via refusal to cooperate, going off fluid & dietary regimens, etc.;

— be aware that weight loss, pallor, loss of energy, shunts, & venipuncture scars are all reminders to pt. that his body integrity is interrupted by illness & Rx, & result in a lessened sense of self; this is often increased by changes in usual role functioning; dialysis pts. can become very attached to "their" machine & incorporate it into their body image;

— help pt. adjust to body image changes by giving recognition for any involvement in planning & managing own care, by eliciting his feelings & listening carefully to what s/he says, & by reminding him of his use of previously successful coping mechanisms for stressful situations; this reaffirmation of his ability to cope will help revive pt.'s good feelings of self;

— provide opportunities for pt. to exert some degree of control over own life, e.g., planning & managing own care via scheduling of Rx, fluids, foods, etc.; involve pt. as much as possible; reassure pt. that increasing independence from the health team is a sign of progress, & not rejection by staff;

— encourage spouse & children to attend a support group, if available, in hospital or community; family members need help in coping with a variety of feelings in relation to the dialysis.

5) Diet and Medications

The patient will develop own menus within dietary restrictions; the patient will adhere to prescribed dietary and medication regimens, and will know the role of each in own treatment:

— acquaint yourself thoroughly with prescribed dietary regimen via unit dietary manual & conferences with dietician; know that they will vary depending on MD, pt.'s blood chemistry levels, local foods available, etc.; see NCPG #3:44, "Diet: Sodium-Restricted;"

— assess pt.'s knowledge of his dietary regimen & ability to select menus; teach PRN & reinforce dietary teaching done by others;

— know, & share with pt. & family, that diet plays a key role in pt.'s struggle to achieve homeostasis; explain restrictions & why they are necessary;

— have pt. keep a chart of own food intake &, if possible, calculate daily ingested amounts of Na, K, protein, fluid, etc.;

— explain actions of medications & their role in controlling pt.'s disease; have pt. make out a list of these & include possible side effects;

— know that a drug regimen can vary widely & depends on many variables such as pt.'s age, condition, extent of disease, etc.; discuss these with MD, pharmacist for specific information, & share with pt. as appropriate;

— *never give an IM injection to pt. during or immediately after hemodialysis* (because these pts. will be heavily heparinized & a severe hematoma can occur); aspirin is usually withheld because it can act as an anticoagulant; acetaminophen can be substituted;

— give dialyzable drugs (e.g., some antibiotics and vitamins) at end of dialysis, for maximum effectiveness;

— hold digitalis preparations until posthemodialysis; hold antihypertensive drugs unless otherwise ordered; check unit protocol & procedures;

— work with the inservice education dept. of your facility to develop teaching aids for pt.

6) Maintenance of AV shunt

The patient will learn to care for own shunt so as to maintain its patency, to prevent infection, and to protect the shunt from injury:

— assess pt.'s knowledge & ability to carry out skin-cleansing technique at shunt site & teach PRN (protocol may vary between facilities);

— assess pt.'s ability to check shunt for patency by palpating the thrill or hearing the bruit in the internal shunt; with the external shunt, check if skin is cool; if there is obvious separation of cells & serum in the shunt & "declotting" is needed, it should be done only by experienced personnel;

— if external shunt is used, teach pt. necessary restrictions for bathing, swimming; ensure s/he has 2 bulldog clamps on self at all times in case of accidental separation of cannulae, & be sure pt. knows how to use them;

— protect shunt from injury; avoid any constriction on arm (e.g., BP cuff, tourniquet, tight clothing); pt. should not carry purse or packages on affected arm; avoid sleeping on arm or other pressures or weights; no routine venipuncture for blood samples, no IV, IM, or SQs in shunt arm;

— teach pt. to check shunt site for swelling, coolness, redness, or other discoloration of skin that might presage an infection or leak in shunt, & to report these to dialysis team.

Discharge Planning and Teaching Objectives/Outcomes

Read this section in NCPG #3:14, "Chronic Renal Failure."

1) (Patient/Family/Significant Other) Knows how to take care of AV shunt in terms of protection from injury, maintenance of patency, prevention of infection, and emergency procedures.

2) Is aware of and can talk about body image changes related to dialysis and dependence for life on a machine.

3) Exerts some control over own life by managing own care, arranging schedules, etc.

4) Has a list of currently prescribed medications, knows dosage schedule, actions, and side effects.

5) (If on home dialysis) Has completed training program, has essential equipment, and is prepared to do dialysis at home.

6) Has appropriate emergency call numbers for doctor and dialysis unit.

Recommended References

Booklets available from Kidney Disease Control Program, National Center for Chronic Disease Control, USPHS, 4040 N. Fairfax Drive, Arlington, VA 22203.

"Complications of Bovine Grafts—Management and Prevention," by D. Aridge. *Nephrology Nurse*, July/August 1981:22–25.

"Diet: Sodium-Restricted." *NCP Guide #3:44*, 2nd Ed., Nurseco, 1983.

"Fluids and Electrolytes, Parts A and B." *NCP Guides #3:48, 49*, 2nd Ed., Nurseco, 1983.

Memory Bank for HemoDialysis, by O. Cairoli and P. Voyce. Pacific Palisades, CA: Nurseco, 1982.

Nephrology for Nurses, 2nd Ed., by J. Cameron and D. Sale. Flushing, NY: Medical Examination Publishing Co., 1976.

Nephrology Nursing, by F. Hekelman and C. Ostendarp. New York: McGraw-Hill, 1979.

Nephrology Nursing Standards of Clinical Practice. Pitman, NJ: American Association of Nephrology Nurses and Technicians (Box 56, 08071), 1982.

"Patient Behaviors." *NCP Guides #1:20–1:33*, 2nd Ed., Nurseco, 1980.

"Patient Education as a Nursing Intervention for Control-Seeking Behaviors," by J. Morris. *Nephrology Nurse*, September/October 1981:20–23.

"The Patient Who is a Kidney Transplant Recipient." *NCP Guide #3:07*, 2nd Ed., Nurseco, 1983.

"Preventing the Spread of Hepatitis B in Dialysis Units," by D. Bauer. *American Journal of Nursing*, February 1980:260–261.

Review of Hemodialysis for Nurses and Dialysis Personnel, 3rd Ed, by C. Gutch and M. Stoner. St. Louis: Mosby, 1979.

"A Review of Hepatitis (Cause & Prevention) for Nephrology Nurses," by A. Corea. *Nephrology Nurse*, May/June 1979:17–22.

The Patient on Hemodialysis: Home

LONG TERM GOAL: The patient will carry out all aspects of own dialysis treatments at home, within the prescribed medical regimen.

General Considerations:

— **Home dialysis** is an excellent treatment modality for maintenance dialysis. Originally all home dialysis was hemodialysis; however some centers are sending patients home with intermittent peritoneal dialysis and a new modality known as Continuous Ambulatory Peritoneal Dialysis (CAPD).

— **Advantages** include economic (the cost is less than ½ the cost of treatment in other centers), convenience (patient can set up a flexible schedule that will accommodate job/school, social life), less risk of medical complications (e.g., hepatitis rate is lower than in hospital dialysis), psychosocial (preservation of family life, greater degree of independence and confidence), and rehabilitation (90% of home dialysis patients are fully rehabilitated, compared with 50% of hospital dialysis patients).

— **The major disadvantages** are disruption of the family schedule and the fact that success or failure depends to a great degree on the personalities of the patient and/or family/significant other (SO). The spouse/SO often feels directly responsible for the life of the patient, with resultant damage to the relationship.

— **Home dialysis is based on three general principles:** (1) chronic disease can be treated better at home than in a hospital; (2) better results will be obtained when the patient is responsible for his own care; and (3) the patient will be better able to care for himself when s/he is well informed of details and complications of his care.

— Review NCPGs #3:03, "Hemodialysis," #3:05, "Peritoneal Dialysis," and #3:14, "Chronic Renal Failure."

— **Nursing responsibilities** include discussion and counseling with patient and family/SO re: feelings, anxieties, frustrations, responsibilities of home dialysis; teaching the patient all aspects of care, including problem solving for potential complications, and reinforcing the role of spouse/SO as that of "helper" rather than "treatment person."

Specific Considerations, Potential Patient Outcomes, and Nursing Actions:

1) Transition to Self Care   The patient will demonstrate ability to initiate, maintain, and terminate dialysis treatment; the patient will demonstrate ability to care for equipment; the patient will maintain fluid and electrolyte balance, will adhere to dietary restrictions, and will take prescribed medications; the patient will show adequate knowledge of problem-solving techniques by correctly answering questions given to him on potential complications and emergencies:

- familiarize yourself with the training program for home dialysis pts. specific to the center from which the pt. is being discharged; these programs usually include essential areas of operation & maintenance of dialysis equipment, purpose & functions of dialysis, self-venipuncture, monitoring & interpreting vital signs, managing complications, ordering supplies, fluid & electrolyte balance, dietary management, & self-medication;
- begin the training program when a decision is made to put pt. on home dialysis; teach pt. one skill at a time, beginning with the simple & proceeding to the complex; assess the pt.'s readiness & ability to learn & proceed at his pace, rather than at yours;
- review NCPGs #1:49 & #1:50, "Teaching Suggestions;" review the teaching program from your center/agency to ensure that it is set up & carried out in a logical, sequential manner;
- expect that pt. will feel discouraged, overwhelmed, inadequate, anxious when "in training;" discuss these feelings with him (unresolved feelings, or feelings that are suppressed & not dealt with, can hinder the learning process); reward pt. for all efforts at expressing & resolving feelings;
- know that pt.'s own motivation is the single most important factor in a successful dialysis program; to foster this, give pt. a great deal of praise & many rewards for learning the essential skills, etc. (research shows that such external rewards are a major way of fostering internal motivation);
- review & reinforce with pt. the principles of fluid & electrolyte balance (NCPGs #3:48 & 49); have him correlate his needs/restrictions with the dialysis, correcting PRN; show pt. how to keep own I&O record;
- ask pt. to tell you about his dietary restrictions; check his menu planning; work with him to find new foods or new ways of preparing old ones that will give him some dietary variety; work with a dietician;
- assess pt.'s self-medication schedule & correct PRN; show him how to keep own med record;
- outline (in depth) complications, (e.g., drop in BP, ruptured dialyzer, line separation, air in lines, infiltrated venipuncture, clotted dialyzer, machine malfunction) & immediate solutions;
- teach pt. the basic steps of problem solving, & explain how s/he can apply them to own dialysis treatment; periodically check his problem-solving ability by posing a potential problem to him & then critique his answer,

correcting PRN; know that problem-solving skills are a high level of cognitive functioning & that you should proceed slowly with pt., reinforcing his ability at each step, & only after he has mastered at least some of the basic skills of the procedure.

2) Psycho-social Adjustment

The patient will learn to identify and discuss emotional feelings related to home hemodialysis; the patient will know what to expect in terms of family disruption;
— know that home dialysis can serve to bring families closer together or can create problems of conflicts, frustration, depression, remorse, withdrawal; much of the success of a home dialysis program depends on the people involved & their ability to deal with stress & long-term illness;
— periodically elicit the feelings of the pt. & discuss these with him; share with pt. that these feelings are usual & expected, & may be intermittent;
— discuss pt.'s participation in a community support group of other dialysis pts. where feelings & problems can be handled on an on-going basis (often this sharing with others in a similar situation can help pt. deal with own feelings); encourage spouse/SO to do the same; if no dialysis group can be found, contact a local mental health center for referrals to other sources;
— reinforce that the role of the spouse/SO is that of "helper" with the dialysis (helps with venipuncture PRN, is available in case of emergency), rather than "doer" (research shows that when spouse/SO assumes too much responsibility, the overall results of home dialysis are poorer); reinforce that the main responsibility for the dialysis rests with the pt.;
— work with the pt. to adjust dialysis schedule to accommodate work & social events, trying to maintain as normal a life as possible;
— know that sexual impotence is a concomitant of chronic renal disease (but dialysis pts. are capable of sexual intercourse); sexual relations can be further hindered because dialysis equipment is usually set up in the bedroom & often the dialysis is done during the night; discuss this area with pt. & spouse/SO; work with them to change schedule, use another physical space if possible, etc.

Discharge Planning and Teaching Objectives/Outcomes

1) (Patient and/or Family/Significant Other) Accepts responsibility for home treatment; can identify feelings and frustrations associated with home dialysis and is able to talk about them with family and nurse.

2) Has initiated, monitored, and terminated dialysis procedure in hospital (center) and plans to do so at home on a continuing basis.

3) Maintains own flow sheet and records, including I&O, diet, and medications.

4) Understands potential dialysis-related complications or emergencies that might occur, and knows how to problem solve to correct them.

5) Has plans to participate in a community support group where s/he can continually deal with feelings and share them with others.

Recommended References

"Assessing the Dialysis Patient at Home," by J. Chambers. *American Journal of Nursing*, April 1981:750–754.

"Evaluation of a Home Hemodialysis Instruction Program," by M. Weiss. *Nephrology Nurse*, July/August 1981:8, 10–12, 42–43.

"Fluids and Electrolytes, Parts A and B." *NCP Guides #3:48, 49*, 2nd Ed., Nurseco, 1983.

"The Home Hemodialysis Assistant: Outpatient Groups," by C. Roy and M. Shurr. *Nephrology Nurse*, September/October 1981:39–44.

Kidney Disease "The Facts," by S. Cameron. New York: Oxford University Press, 1981.

"The Patient in Renal Failure: Chronic." *NCP Guide #3:14*, 2nd Ed., Nurseco, 1983.

"The Patient on Dialysis: Hemodialysis." *NCP Guide #3:03*, 2nd Ed., Nurseco, 1983.

"The Patient on Dialysis: Peritoneal." *NCP Guide #3:05*, 2nd Ed., Nurseco, 1983.

Replacement of Renal Function by Dialysis, by W. Drukker, E. Parson, and J.H. Maker. Boston: Martinus Nijhoff Medical, 1978.

Strategy in Renal Failure, by E. Friedman Eli. New York: Wiley, 1978.

"Teaching Patients: General Suggestions." *NCP Guide #1:49*, 2nd Ed., Nurseco, 1980.

"Teaching Patients: Specific Plan for Skills and Procedures." *NCP Guide #1:50*, 2nd Ed., Nurseco, 1980.

"Teaching Young Patients—and their Families—about Home Peritoneal Dialysis," by S. Gross. *Nursing 80*, December 1980:72–73.

Understanding Your New Life with Dialysis, by E. Oberley and T. Oberley. Springfield, IL: Charles Thomas, 1975.

The Patient on Dialysis: Peritoneal

Definition: The diffusion of solute molecules through a semipermeable membrane (the peritoneum) from the side of higher concentration to that of the lower concentration.

LONG TERM GOAL: The patient will adhere to prescribed regimen to aid recovery from the acute renal failure and to return to usual roles; OR—the patient will adapt to the reality of long-term dialysis and will live within its accompanying limitations.

General Considerations:
— Read this section in NCPG #3:03, "The Patient on Dialysis: Hemodialysis."
— **How does it work?** Peritoneal dialysis (PD) is based on two principles: (1) *diffusion*, wherein molecules and ions of accumulated wastes and toxins pass from an area of higher concentration (the patient's blood) to that of a lower concentration (the dialysate); and (2) *osmosis*, the diffusion of a solution through a semipermeable membrane (the peritoneum). Thus a high concentration of solutes in the patient's blood will move through the peritoneum into the dialysate in the peritoneal cavity. The dialysate is removed repetitively and replaced with fresh solution in order to maintain a high mean diffusion gradient between body fluids and dialysate.
— **Procedure:**
a) *access*: insertion of a catheter into the peritoneal cavity is carried out by a doctor under strict aseptic technique (signed operative permit necessary). The catheter used in acute PD is made of teflon and is removed following the PD treatment; for chronic PD, the catheter is made of silastic with a dacron felt cuff (bacterial barrier) and has an average life of nine months.
b) *Dialysis is accomplished by repeating a three-phase cycle.* Each cycle includes (1) inflow (the time it takes to flow dialysate into the peritoneal cavity), (2) diffusion or dialysis (the time that the dialysate is in contact with the peritoneal cavity), and (3) outflow (the time it takes the dialysate to drain from the peritoneal cavity).
c) *Method*:
• *manual single bottle method*: the catheter is attached to Y-tubing and prescribed fluid (usually one to two liters of sterile dialyzing solution *warmed to body temperature*) is run in by gravity (10–15 minutes); the tubing is clamped just before the bottles or bags are empty (inflow phase); the dialysate remains in the peritoneal cavity for 30–40 minutes until a degree of equilibrium between the dialysate and body fluids is achieved (diffusion or dialysis phase); the bottles or bags are lowered to the floor, the tubing unclamped, and the fluid drains out over 15–20 minutes (outflow phase).

- *automatic PD system*: a machine composes, sterilizes, and cycles the dialysate through the three phases (monitors and alarms are incorporated into the system). In either the manual or automatic method, the fluid exchange is repeated until blood chemistries are nearing normal, usually 36–48 hours (30–40 exchanges), and may be done as often as three times/week.
- *Continuous Ambulatory Peritoneal Dialysis* (CAPD) is achieved by completing three to five cycles/day, seven days/week. A prescribed amount of dialysate is connected to the permanent catheter, allowed to gravity flow into the abdomen (inflow phase), then clamped and allowed to dwell (diffusion or dialysis phase) for four to five hours. During this time the empty dialysate bag is folded and the patient carries it around with him. After diffusion, the empty dialysate bag is dropped to a clean surface (usually a paper towel on the floor), unclamped, and the dialysate is allowed to gravity flow out (outflow phase). The process is then repeated with new dialysate. The evening cycle is allowed to dwell (diffusion or dialysis phase) seven to eight hours at night.
- *Continuous Cycling Peritoneal Dialysis* (CCPD) is a treatment that is basically a reversal of CAPD exchanges. CAPD is normally done during the day with the long dwell (diffusion or dialysis phase) during the night. CCPD does cycles during the night with a simple cycling machine, and the long dwell (diffusion or dialysis phase) during the day. This type of treatment affords the patient much more personal freedom for day activity.
— **Nursing responsibilities** are primarily those of assembling and setting up equipment, providing physical and emotional comfort to patient, and observing for and detecting early signs and symptoms of impending or potential complications.

Specific Considerations, Potential Patient Outcomes, and Nursing Actions:

1) Preparation of Patient

The patient will know what to expect in terms of length of procedure, discomfort, oral intake; the patient will be involved in planning own care, when feasible, to achieve physical and emotional comfort:
- — assess pt.'s knowledge of procedure & provide as much information as s/he requests & needs to know; speak in calm, reassuring tones; let pt. know how long & at what times a nurse will be at pt.'s side;
- — plan care with pt., involving him as much as possible; if s/he has been dialyzed previously, ask what you can do to enhance comfort during this dialysis;
- — assemble all equipment & solutions & read manufacturers' labels on them; explain each step of procedure to pt.; answer all questions as honestly as you can;
- — assess for restlessness & give meds as ordered;

— provide frequent back rubs, massage pressure areas, & change position PRN (during infusion, pt. is usually supine with head slightly elevated to decrease discomfort of the abdominal organs pushing up against the diaphragm);

— before procedure begins, take (& record on flow sheet) BP, TPR; have pt. empty bladder; assess for headaches, dizziness, etc.

2) Fluids

The patient will experience a smooth fluid exchange; the patient will maintain an adequate fluid balance:

— weigh pt. before & after dialysis & record;

— assess & record pt.'s hydration status by analyzing weight, skin turgor, thirst, mucus membrane moisture, I&O, & edema;

— keep an accurate recording of patient's fluid exchange balance; *for each exchange*, record essential exchange times on flow sheet: (1) time infusion started & (2) ended; (3) time outflow begins & (4) ends;

— record amt. of solutions infused & returned & compute balance, usually a plus or minus amt.;

— if fluid does not drain in a steady stream, apply firm pressure to lower abdomen & ask pt. to turn from side to side;

— check with MD regarding amt. of oral fluids permitted; keep an accurate I&O record;

— describe & record dialysate color & clarity; carefully report any cloudy bags to MD.

3) Prevention of Compli- cations

The patient will be free of preventable complications or, if occurring, will have them promptly detected and optimally managed:

— report to MD & chart any signs or symptoms that are deviations from normal; know that common complications, observations, & critical care include:

  • *shock*: may occur due to excessive fluid loss or overhydration; take BP, P, & R Q15 minutes for 1st hour or until stable, then Q1–2H; if a sudden drop in BP occurs, drain the peritoneal cavity & notify MD *STAT* (hypotension is the most important obstacle to a smooth dialysis);

  • *bleeding*: outflow is usually straw-colored; if active bleeding suspected, notify MD; slight bleeding around acute catheter site may occur; if it continues, notify MD; change dressing around catheter PRN, using strict aseptic technique;

  • *severe abdominal pain*: most often occurs at end of inflow or outflow period; may be caused by (1) dialysate not being at body temperature, (2) incomplete drainage of solution, or (3) may be forewarning of peritoneal infection; procaine 0.5% is sometimes put through tubing immediately before each infusion; check with MD;

- *infection*: risk is high because abdominal catheter acts as a foreign body; strict aseptic technique is mandatory for prevention; chronic catheter must be evaluated for tunnel & exit site infection;
- *draining problems* (main cause of catheter draining problem is constipation): reposition pt., roll side to side, making sure the tubing is not kinked; lower bag or raise pt. higher for more gravity; if all remedies fail to promote drainage, give pt. warm soap & water enema per MD orders;
— if machines are used, monitor equipment throughout dialysis for patency of tubing, temperature of dialysate, security of connections, dialysate conductivity, etc.

4) Psycho-social Adjustment (to Loss of Independence)

The patient will experience only minimum anxiety or fear during procedure; patient will progress in adapting to his dependence on long-term dialysis as a life-maintaining measure:
— remember that dialysis will make the pt. feel better, but not well;
— when pt. returns for continuing dialysis, assess affect & mental status before dialysis; know that a dependence on the health team is established & that pt. may respond with a variety of feelings, all of which can be considered adaptive except suicidal ones; read NCPGs #3:14, "Chronic Renal Failure" (part 4 on Psychosocial Adjustment), and #s1:20–33, "Patient Behaviors;"
— accept stage of grief the pt. is experiencing; accept behavior & encourage pt. to talk about feelings; if anger is displayed to nurse, reflect feelings for pt. ("You seem very angry today.") to help pt. talk about the feelings;
— be aware that asking questions about the procedure & necessary life-style changes is a sign of adaptation by pt.; when this occurs, it is important for the nurse to provide information to pt. & work with him to bring about changes;
— provide diversional activities during dialysis.

5) Health Teaching

The patient will verbalize aspects of prescribed health regimen; the patient will comply with imposed regimen:
— (if pt. on long-term dialysis) periodically review prescribed regimens with pt. & assess degree of compliance; praise for all positive efforts & discuss areas for improvement;
— do not chide for shortcomings; listen to pt.'s explanations, problems, & feelings; work out solutions with pt.; consult social worker, clergy, or mental health worker PRN;
— review foods allowed on diet & health teach PRN;
— review reasons for infection, prevention measures; assess understanding of & compliance with these aspects;
— review NCPGs #1:49 & #1:50, "Teaching Patients," for educational principles in health teaching.

Discharge Planning and Teaching Objectives/Outcomes
Refer to this section in NCP Guide #3:14, "Chronic Renal Failure."
1) (Patient/Family/Significant Other) Knows that a variety of feelings and emotions are usual and expected in the adaptation process.
2) Is aware of and can accept dependency on health team to keep self alive.
3) If patient goes home with chronic catheter, knows catheter care and dialysis center protocol.
4) Is aware of all potential complications, has telephone number of MD and dialysis center, and knows when to call.

Recommended References
CAPD Update, by J. Moncrief and R. Popovich. New York: Masson, 1981.
"Caring for the Catheter Carefully . . . Before, During, and After Peritoneal Dialysis," by R. Lavandew and V. Davis. *Nursing 80*, November 1980:73–79.
"The Evolution of CAPD," by M. Sandeval and C. Parks. *Nephrology Nurse*, September/October 1981:27, 30, 32.
Nephrology Nursing Standards of Clinical Practice. Pitman, NJ: American Association of Nephrology Nurses and Technicians, 1982.
"Now—Peritoneal Dialysis for Chronic Patients, Too," by B. Irwin. *RN*, June 1981:49–52, 98.
"Open Forum: Peritoneal Dialysis," by R. Oreopoulos et al. *Dialysis and Transplation*, August 1982:663–680.
"The Patient with Renal Failure: Chronic." *NCP Guide #3:14*, 2nd Ed., Nurseco, 1983.
Peritoneal Dialysis, by P. Atkins, N. Thomson, and P. Farrell. New York: Churchill Livingstone, 1981.
"Peritoneal Dialysis: A Rediscovery," by P. Sorrel. *Nursing Clinics of North America*, September 1981:515–529.
"Responses to Loss: The Grief and Mourning Process." *NCP Guide #1:31*, 2nd Ed., Nurseco, 1980.
"Teaching Patients: General Suggestions." *NCP Guide #1:49*, 2nd Ed., Nurseco, 1980.
"Teaching Patients: Specific Plan for Skills and Procedures." *NCP Guide #1:50*, 2nd Ed., Nurseco, 1980.

The Patient with Epilepsy

Definition: Epilepsy is a disorder of the nervous system, characterized by sudden and periodic lapses of consciousness known as seizures. The electrical disturbance of the brain may be caused by a single factor, a combination of factors, or be unknown.

LONG TERM GOAL: The patient will lead a relatively normal life assuming family and community roles/responsibilities; the patient will be seizure-free due to continuing medication and avoidance of precipitating stimuli; the patient will understand and accept the reality of a probably lifetime condition and will cope effectively with society's rejection and lack of understanding.

General Considerations:
— **Incidence:** approximately 1% of general American population; estimates vary because victims often "hide" symptoms or diagnosis.
— **Occurrence:** both sexes, any age or race.
— **Seizure classification** (international):
  • **Partial Seizures** (local onset)
     a) *Partial with elementary symptomatology* includes focal motor (Jacksonian or one-sided progression) jerking, focal sensory symptoms (numbness, coldness, tingling, illusions of olfactory, gustatory, visual, or auditory sensations), or autonomic symptoms (tachycardia, flushing, diaphoresis, blood pressure changes); area of convulsion or sensation depends on localized area of brain that is over-active, stimulated, or damaged.
     b) *Partial with complex symptomatology*, also known as psychomotor or temporal lobe seizures; consists of pre-seizure aura (any combination of cognitive, affective, sensory, or psychomotor symptoms), altered state of consciousness and a variety of purposeless behaviors such as chewing, lip smacking, picking at clothes, rubbing arms or legs, feelings of fear or anxiety, confusion or dizziness, pain, buzzing or ringing in ears, etc.; after seizure, there is no memory of what happened.
  • **Generalized Seizures** (symmetrical without local onset) including (but not limited to):
     a) *Absence seizures*, also known as petit mal, involves a lapse of attention similar to day-dreaming or blank staring (with possible eye fluttering) that may last a few seconds to less than a minute. After this loss of contact with the environment, individual's activity continues as if nothing had happened.

    b) *Tonic-clonic seizures*, also known as grand mal, consists of loss of consciousness, a rigid posture phase, followed by bilateral rhythmic violent jerking movements of face, eyes, neck, trunk, and limbs. Saliva-drooling and noisy, labored breathing are common; cyanosis and incontinence may occur. Convulsion may last one to three minutes or longer and may be followed by period of confusion, speech difficulty, headache, weakness, fatigue, and drowsiness leading to deep sleep.

— **Diagnosis** is made via a thorough history, complete physical and neurological examination with a battery of tests including skull x-rays, brain scan, angiography, pneumoencephalogram, and EEG (electroencephalogram). See Recommended References to prepare patient for an EEG.

— **Treatment** aim is to control or minimize seizures via medication; to remove or control any known causes of seizure activity; and to establish good general health with a balanced, moderate, fairly normal, and active lifestyle. Restrictions re: operating vehicles or machinery will be determined by state laws and physician according to patient's seizure-free record. Surgery is indicated only in a small percentage (5%) of patients under select situations (single focal seizure area that is surgically accessible, unresponsiveness to intensive drug therapy, and probability of overall improvement of patient's existence).

— **Nursing responsibilities** include assistance with diagnosis and treatment plan; seizure precautions and prevention of injury; patient/ family/significant other (SO) education and counseling re: reality of epilepsy, acceptance and compliance with continuing medical regimen, preparation to assume self-confident self-care; and public education to abate misconceptions, prejudice, and fear of epileptics in society. Epilepsy clinical nurse specialists are now available and may be consulted for nursing staff development and community education programs.

Specific Considerations, Potential Patient Outcomes, and Nursing Actions:

1) Seizure Precautions and Care

The patient will be free of injuries and will not aspirate tongue, mucus, or foreign objects; the patient's seizure will be controlled as safely and as soon as possible; the patient's seizures will be accurately observed, described, and documented; the patient will regain postictal orientation and stable condition;

— keep bed rails up & padded when pt. is in bed; explain to pt. & gain acceptance;

— check pt.'s vital signs & level of consciousness Q2H; observe & report unusual behavior:

— tape plastic oral airway in one clearly designated, easily accessible place (usually head of bed) & have an alternate on the pt. when s/he leaves room for diagnostic tests, meals, or other reasons;

— label all x-ray, lab, & off-nursing unit situation requests with "Seizure Precautions" in red ink;

— hold conferences for nursing staff, auxiliary medical personnel, & pt.'s family/friends re: this pt.'s particular type of seizure (once it has been fully described & identified) & the safe, appropriate first aid care measures to be provided;

— supervise pt. showers & smoking;

— take only rectal or axillary temperatures & notify all nursing staff of this precautionary measure;

— have accessible for immediate use: oxygen & suction equipment, IV supplies, parenteral antiepileptic drugs (more than one type—diazepam, phenobarbital, & phenytoin), cardiac & respiratory stimulants, & IV bicarbonate;

— never leave pt. alone once a seizure begins; if possible, put pt. in supine, side-lying position; loosen clothing at neck & waist; remove glasses; protect head with your arms, lap, cushion, or safe substitute; protect pt. from environmental dangers (furniture, walls, equipment);

— for complex partial seizures, do not try to stop purposeless behavior & do not touch, annoy or argue with pt. out of control; urge onlookers to leave scene, assuring them that you will cope with situation;

— for semi- or unconscious pts., establish an open airway with head position (extended neck, face turned to side) if possible & intubation airway if available; place folded towel, padded tongue blade or other safe substitute between teeth at side of mouth, if possible, but *do not force open* clenched teeth; suction secretions PRN;

— remain with pt. until fully conscious & reoriented or until you have determined pt. to be in stable postictal condition, although asleep; check vital signs; when possible, reorient pt. to name, time, place, & surroundings; explain what happened; be calm & reassuring; speak slowly, comfort witnesses;

— record observations in chronological sequence: time, onset of unusual behavior, environmental stimulants or other possible pre-seizure factors (photosensitivity, chill, fatigue, stressors), description of ictal phase, location & type of tonic or clonic contractions, presence of incontinence, skin color & condition, automisms (eye fluttering, lip smacking), eye movements & pupillary changes, duration of seizure, description of postictal phase & progress of pt.'s condition, sensorium, level of awareness, speech difficulty, weakness, pain, & length of time it takes for pt. to be reoriented & stabilized;

— teach nursing staff & family/SO how to accurately observe & describe seizures;

— notify physician STAT if seizures are repetitive without periods of consciousness or if seizure lasts longer than 30 minutes; know emergency protocol for status epilepticus (SE); prepare to start (& keep open) IV fluids with anti-epileptic drugs (usually quick-acting diazepam to start); monitor frequently the prescribed slow infusion rate; observe closely for respiratory & cardiac depression; maintain adequate oxygenation to prevent hypoxia; suction pharynx frequently & PRN; monitor vital signs Q15 minutes & PRN; initiate I&O records; prepare to administer hypothermia measures PRN; arrange for transfer to intensive care unit or provide 1-to-1 nursing observation & care; know that EEG monitoring may be needed to differentiate SE-related from non-convulsive (stuporous) type seizures so that appropriate, effective antiepileptic drug can be selected;

— after an episode of SE, observe (& take control measures) for fever, diaphoresis, hypertension; assist MD to discover SE precipitant; know that these include withdrawal from alcohol, sedatives, or antiepileptic drugs; fever, trauma, intoxication, & sleep deprivation;

— teach pt./family/SO that seizure threshold can be lowered still further by factors such as malnutrition, fatigue, infection, injury, psychological stress, alcohol or drug abuse, menstruation, pregnancy, body weight changes, & sudden life changes; help pt. plan a living style that recognizes, prevents, or controls these factors; refer PRN to NCPG #5:49, "Stress Management."

2) Medications   The patient will comply with drug regimen; the patient will state the importance of taking medication regularly to prevent seizures; the patient will help identify symptoms of toxic effects by reporting regularly to nurse or physician how s/he feels and when s/he notices anything different in reactions:

— explain to pt./family/SO all necessary information about each medication (name, dosage, frequency, toxic & side effects to observe & report);

— emphasize the necessity of maintaining a therapeutic blood level by not missing or postponing doses; have a clear understanding from MD what is to be done for a missed dose;

— know that epileptics commonly feel an intense dislike for drugs that make them feel "doped up;" explore resentment & work through to acceptance level;

— recommend to pt. to take antiepileptic drugs with meals or large quantities of water to minimize gastrointestinal disturbances;

— monitor vital signs Q2H during first 3 days of new drug regimen;

— know, observe, record, & report promptly side & toxic effects of antiepileptic drugs (drowsiness, dizziness, rash, gastric distress, vision problems, hyperexcitability, confusion, muscular incoordination);

— know that pts. on Dilantin & phenobarbital may have calcium & Vit. D deficiencies; give calcium supplements if ordered & observe for pathological fractures related to osteomalacia;

— know that phenytoin (Dilantin) blood levels can increase when pt. is on other drugs (alcohol, anti-coagulants, Antabuse, isoniazid) or when pt. is having an illness that affects liver or kidney function; observe & report increased incidence of toxic effects;

— know that other drugs may interact negatively with antiepileptic drugs (aspirin, narcotics, folic acid, & certain antibiotics); antacids may interfere with absorption & proper blood levels of antiepileptic drugs;

— emphasize & teach meticulous oral hygiene with flossing, since gum enlargement (gingival hyperplasia) is associated with long-term phenytoin usage;

— teach effective skin cleansing with anti-acne products, since antiepileptic drugs contribute to a worsening acne problem.

3) Psycho-
   logical
   Adjustment

The patient will verbalize feelings, fears, anxieties related to diagnosis; the patient will understand and accept the reality of own condition and try to live a normal, self-confident, independent life; the patient will strive to maintain a positive self-concept; the patient will cope with the negative attitudes of non-epileptics:

— promote & facilitate an open discussion of feelings, attitudes, & beliefs between pt., family & nurse or MD; bring out questions, misconceptions, fears, & the reality of public discrimination or social stigma of epilepsy; know that the common psychological problem behaviors include anxiety, denial, guilt, depression, withdrawal, low self-esteem, hostility, & aggression, among others;

— know that emotional stress can lower seizure threshold; discuss with pt. & family their current coping mechanisms & possible new ones:

— supply literature from local & national epilepsy organizations; read & clarify these with family/SO;

— encourage participation in mutual support groups of fellow epileptics;

— respect pt.'s decision to conceal condition, but insist on some identification (disease, doctor, meds) being kept on person & on file in school or employment medical records;

— review with pt./family/SO problems of living arrangements, employment, insurance, auto driving, & operating dangerous machinery; know that state laws differ; refer to State Bureaus of Vocational Rehabilitation, Developmental Disabilities, or Human Resources for information & help;

— refer to local office of US Dept. of Labor or State Human Rights Commission for issues of job discrimination (prohibited by 1973 Federal Rehabilitation Act protecting handicapped).

Discharge Planning and Teaching Objectives/Outcomes

1) (Patient/Family/Significant Other) Can state basic facts of epilepsy with relevance to own condition.
2) Can name own pre-seizure symptoms and what to do for own type of seizure.
3) States knowledge of potential seizure triggers and how they can be avoided or minimized.
4) Knows all prescribed medications (name, dosage, frequency of administration, side & toxic effects); has a written copy of this information; indicates a willingness to comply with drug regimen; has an acceptable plan for medication storage, refills, and missed dosage.
5) States s/he understands necessity for regular follow-up doctor visits while on anticonvulsive therapy, even though seizure-free; promises to report promptly to MD with possible pregnancy, body weight changes, life style changes, signs of illness (fever, infection), injuries to head, or when involved in other crisis situations (loss of loved one, etc.).
6) Expresses familiarity with services of Epilepsy Foundation of America (and local affiliates); has at least one of its publications along with the name and address of the nearest chapter.
7) Wears a Medic-Alert (or AMA Emergency) identification object and carries an ID card in wallet with information re: condition, medications, doctor name and number.

Recommended References

"Identification and Treatment of Status Epilepticus," by Mary Pat Lovely. *Journal of Neurosurgical Nursing*, June 1980:93-96.

A Patient's Guide to EEG-Electroencephalography, Medications for Epilepsy, The Role of Nurse in the Understanding and Treatment of Epilepsy (and other literature for parents, patients, and professionals). Landover, MD: Epilepsy Foundation of America (4351 Garden City Drive, 20785).

"Psychosocial Aspects of Epilepsy," by Judy Ozuna. *Journal of Neurosurgical Nursing*, December 1979:242-246.

"Seizure Disorders," by Susan Norman and Thomas Browne. "Nursing Management," and "Surgical Treatment of Epilepsy," by Susan Norman. "Complex Partial Seizures," by Catherine Tucker. *The American Journal of Nursing*, May 1981:984-1000.

"Stress Management." *NCP Guide #5:49*, Nurseco, 1981.

"The Reality of Epilepsy," by Judy Beniak et al. *The Journal of Practical Nursing*, March 1980:22-26, 38.

The Patient who is a Kidney Transplant Recipient

LONG TERM GOAL: The patient will adjust and adhere to a life-long, limited medical regimen imposed by the kidney transplant.

General Considerations:
— Kidney transplantation is the ultimate desirable form of treatment for end stage renal disease (ESRD) and provides an alternative to dialysis with its increasing requirements, financial restraints, and quality control.
— The biggest **advantages** are that it allows the patient to return to an almost normal life, releases a dialysis bed for another patient, and eliminates the high cost of dialysis.
— **Donor kidneys** are obtained from either a live donor (better results) or a cadaver. Most potential kidney recipients put in a period of waiting because of a lack of suitable and available kidneys. Seventy percent must await a cadaver transplant because they do not have a relative willing or able to donate one.
— **Tissue typing** must be done pre-op to ensure a transplant as histocompatible as possible. The highest degree of compatibility is with identical twins, then with a sibling, then parent, and lastly with a non-relative. The transplant (allograft) acts as a foreign body within the recipient, thus stimulating the antigen-antibody reaction, leading to rejection.
— The **greatest problem is rejection** (the patient takes high doses of steroids in an effort to prevent rejection of the transplant). Types of rejection: (1) *hyper-acute rejection* happens on the operating room table; the kidney turns black. (2) *Acute rejection* usually happens within the first year post-op. (3) *Chronic rejection* happens despite repeated efforts to increase immuno-suppression; the rejection continues. A patient can survive several bouts of acute rejection, but once chronic rejection begins, it can be an insidious, irreversible process with resultant loss of the transplant. About 60–70% of cadaver donors and 80–90% of live, related donors are not rejected.
— **Decision to transplant** is often based on patient's own wishes, age, whether s/he wants to take the 60-70% chance of a successful transplant, other complications of ESRD, and on how well s/he tolerates and is doing on dialysis.
— **Pre-op management** is required to put the patient in as normal a metabolic state as possible via dialysis, dietary measures, and (sometimes) surgery. It includes eliminating potential sources of post-op infection (extraction of carious teeth, removal of infected kidneys in those with chronic pyelonephritis or polycystic disease). Bilateral nephrectomies are sometimes done to control malignant hypertension that does not respond to dialysis control. However, after bilateral nephrectomies, the patient requires multiple blood transfusions, making this treatment less favorable for uncontrolled hypertension.

— **Treatment** goals are to keep the patient and the transplanted kidney alive and functioning and to prevent infection. The major post-op complications of rejection and infection usually do not appear in the immediate post-op period, but within the first post-op month. Mortality rate is 4–5% and is usually due to sepsis.

— **Nursing responsibilities** include being knowledgeable of the protocol in your facility for the pre- and post-op management of kidney transplant patients; monitoring, maintaining, and supporting the patient in the hospital; and health teaching the patient/family/significant other (SO) for maintenance at home.

Specific Considerations, Potential Patient Outcomes, and Nursing Actions:

1) Pre-op Care   The patient will experience no more than moderate anxiety and will be given as much information as s/he wants & needs to know about the procedure and care; the patient will achieve and maintain fluid balance; the patient will be maintained in an infection-free state:

— ask pt. *what it feels like* now that s/he is finally approaching the reality of receiving a new kidney (usual feelings include euphoria, moderate apprehension & anxiety, fear of failure); share with pt. that these feelings are commonly experienced by others in same situation, & are normal & expected; know that the pt. needs you to help him sort out, interpret, & cope with the many feelings, concerns & questions that burden him;

— assess what pt. *already knows* about the surgery & what s/he *wants* & *needs* to know; teach PRN; be sure pt. demonstrates turning, deep breathing, effective coughing, use of pillow splint; usual questions revolve around potential for rejection of transplant, the shunt, the donor, the need for dialysis post-op, drugs, radiation, limited isolation, overview of surgical day, pain & discomfort; be aware that these pts. are usually much better informed of all the ramifications of their condition than most surgical pts. & tend to ask more questions; be honest; keep your knowledge current;

— maintain an accurate I&O record, including daily weights; adhere to fluid restrictions as ordered by MD (usual is to replace daily loss + 500 ml); hemodialysis may be needed pre-op to stabilize pt. for surgery;

— provide diet strictly as ordered; strict adherence is needed to achieve pre-op metabolic stability;

— use strict hand-washing technique & do not approach pt. if you have any signs of a cold; screen other hospital staff & visitors accordingly; know & carry out other measures for infection control as dictated by protocol of your facility.

2) Post-op
Care and
Prevention
of Compli-
cations

The patient will receive close monitoring during immediate and subsequent post-op periods; the patient will remain free of preventable complications, e.g., atelectasis, shock, blocked urinary drainage, fluid imbalance, infection, others:

— know & carry out post-op orders as dictated by surgeon & unit protocol;
— monitor vital signs, including CVP, & report any changes to MD;
— maintain accurate I&O & record; give fluids only as ordered;
— measure urinary output carefully & accurately; know that pt. may have a *massive diuresis* (especially if transplant is from a live donor), be *anuric* (especially if a cadaver transplant), or have an *output between these two extremes*; keep Foley catheter patent; if necessary to irrigate catheter, do *only* on MD's order, using *strict* aseptic technique; refer to NCPG #2:39, "Catheters;"
— assess fluid balance, considering I&O, daily weight, lab reports, CVP, & pt. status; review NCPG #3:48, "Fluids & Electrolytes;" when pt. able, teach to record own I&O, as preparation for discharge;
— turn, cough, & deep breathe PRN; try to medicate ½ hour before this procedure, & use a pillow splint over incision (as efforts to minimize pain & discomfort); pt. usually positioned on back or operative side; may be ambulatory first PO day, per MD's orders;
— carry out limited isolation techniques (reverse or regular) as dictated by unit protocol; wash hands thoroughly before approaching pt.; screen out all contacts with signs of a cold; take temp Q4H & PRN; know that PO infection often appears within first month;
— observe pt. for signs of acute rejection of kidney transplant (fever, inc. BP, swollen tender kidney, dec. urine volume, & wt. gain); pt. may state that s/he feels s/he's getting the flu; report to MD PRN;
— know that pt. may require temporary post-op dialysis, especially if s/he has a cadaver kidney, to sustain him until the transplant is functioning adequately (may be up to 7 weeks);
— check shunt or fistula frequently for patency (there is a high incidence of thrombosis post-op); shunt should have an even pink color, no blood separation, & should feel warm; an A-V fistula should have a bruit; if any problems, notify MD; these vascular accesses need to be maintained in case pt. needs dialysis; do *not* take BP in shunt arm; do *not* use fistula for blood samples; a shunt can usually be used for blood samples, but under strict aseptic technique;

— observe pt. for signs of hyperkalemia; may develop a high K because of blood transfusions combined with inadequate renal excretion; monitor serum K level at least Q4H; refer to NCPG #2:48, "Potassium Imbalance;"
— monitor acid-base balance; some base deficit will be present but the pH should not fall below 7.4 (check with MD); see NCPG #3:40, "Acid-Base Balance;"
— ambulate pt. ASAP & frequently (helps to lessen post-op complications & effects of muscle wasting due to steroids).

3) Medications   The patient will learn to take own immuno-suppressive medications and will keep a written schedule of ingestion:
— know (& reinforce to pt.) that these drugs are the main defense against rejection of the transplant; consult a PDR or the literature accompanying the drugs for specific information on each one; be aware of interactions & complications; warn pt. that severe rejection &/or death may happen if immuno-suppressive drugs are stopped suddenly;
— maintain accurate medication records; give meds only as ordered or per unit protocol;
— assess pt's. knowledge of drugs s/he is taking, their effect, possible side effects, etc.; teach PRN;
— teach pt. to self-medicate & to keep a med record, both *in hospital* & after discharge;
— know (& reinforce to pt.) that the immuno-suppressive drugs suppress the body's ability to cope with infection; teach pt. strict infection control measures; when s/he is ready, discuss ways pt./family/SO can carry out infection control at home; share with pt. that as the drug dosage is decreased, the body slowly learns to cope with some degree of infection; tell pt. to contact MD at first sign of a cold.

4) Psycho-   The patient will experience minimal post-op anxiety; the patient will learn to cope with the possibilities of post-op
   social   infection, rejection, dialysis, and with feelings of euphoria, depression, etc.:
   Adjustment   — because these pts. are usually well-informed, they may want to know their urinary output, vital signs, lab results, status of shunt, etc.; give them as much info. as they want, pointing out the positive signs; inform them of status of the live, related donor; be aware that providing info. a pt. wants is a major way of decreasing anxiety;
— assess if pt. wants to discuss potential post-op complications; if so, do it in an open, honest manner, answering all questions;

— reassure pt. that a kidney can experience several bouts of acute rejection & still function, due to its remarkable ability to recover from insult;
— reassure pt. that feelings of euphoria & depression often result from taking steroids, & that they will be short-lived; help pt. to express his feelings to you & to his family, & to discuss them together as a way of dealing with them;
— when pt. is ready, discuss discharge plans & ways to control infection, medication, & diet at home; work with both pt. family/significant others.

Discharge Planning and Teaching Objectives/Outcomes

1) (Patient/Family/Significant Other) Has a list of medications with dosage and schedule; knows side effects of each, the importance of adhering to prescribed dosages, and knows where and how to obtain refills; can keep own medication record.
2) Can maintain own I&O record; knows food and fluid restrictions and is able to plan daily menus and intake accordingly.
3) Can verbalize current feelings and anxieties and knows that they are usual and expected; has a referral and/or appointment with a community support group, mental health clinic, etc.
4) Has appointment for return visit to transplant clinic/doctor.

Recommended References

"Acid-Base Balance." *NCP Guide #3:40*, 2nd Ed., Nurseco, 1983.
"Catheters: Indwelling Urinary." *NCP Guide #2:39*, 2nd Ed., Nurseco, 1980.
"Chronic Renal Disease in Children," by M. Topor. *Nursing Clinics of North America*, September 1981:587–597.
"Fluids and Electrolytes, Parts A and B." *NCP Guides #3:48, 49*, 2nd Ed., Nurseco, 1983.
"From One Death, Two Lives," by E. Monroe. *AORN Journal*, October 1974:613–617.
Nephrology Nursing Standards of Clinical Practice. Pitman, NJ: American Association of Nephrology Nurses and Technichians (Box 56, 08071), 1982.
"Potassium Imbalance." *NCP Guide #2:48*, 2nd Ed., Nurseco, 1980.
"Renal Transplantation," by J. Cianci, J. Lamp, and R. Ryan. *American Journal of Nursing*, February 1981:354–355.
Renal Transplantation, a Nursing Perspective, by B. Sachs. Flushing, NY: Medical Examination Publishing Co., 1977.
"Renal Transplantation: The Patient's Choice," by A. Powers. *Nursing Clinics of North America*, September 1981:551–564.
Nephrology Nurse (whole issue on transplantation). November/December 1981.
"What Patients Awaiting Kidney Transplant Want to Know," by Z. Wolf. *American Journal of Nursing*, January 1976:92–94.

The Patient with a Laminectomy/Spinal Fusion/Discectomy

Definition: *Micro/macro discectomy* is the excision of displaced intervertebral disc (or disk) material. *Laminectomy* is the removal of the spinous processes and lamina above and below the affected disc in order to remove the protruding disc material that is pressing on the spinal nerves. (Laminectomies may also be done for cord tumors or fractured spines.) *Spinal fusion* is the union of two or three vertebral surfaces in order to stabilize movement of a joint where abnormal motion of this unstable segment has contributed to the pain.

LONG TERM GOAL: The patient will recover from back surgery free of preventable complications, returning to home/family/community roles and responsibilities while adapting to a regimen of back care appropriate to improved health status and rehabilitation.

General Considerations:
— **Incidence:** more than 200,000 laminectomies are done yearly; microdiscectomies are replacing conventional macrosurgical approaches in selected patients for first time disc surgery at affected level. The microsurgical operation is done through a one-inch incision, involves less soft tissue disruption and pain, a shorter recovery period, and a more satisfactory rehabilitation to former activity levels.

— **Diagnosis:** a thorough history and physical showing positive neurological signs, significant straight leg raising deficit, signs of involved nerve root irritation, and sciatica (leg pain). Positive findings are confirmed with myelogram, EMG, and CT Scan.

— **Myelogram** (x-ray of the spinal cord after aqueous contrast medium is injected into the spinal canal) reveals the relationship of the disc to nerve root and the degree of nerve root compression. The nurse and physician should explain the procedure to the patient in careful detail. Myths and misconceptions must be corrected and every attempt made to allay the patient's heightened sense of anxiety. Phenobarbital is given before and after water-soluble Metrazide-medium myelograms to prevent rare side effect of seizures. Other sedative/analgesic/muscle relaxant medications may be given to sedate and relax the patient. After the myelogram, the patient remains on bed rest for 24 hours with fluids forced to decrease the chances of post-puncture headaches, back pain, and muscle spasms. Since false positives and false negatives do sometimes occur, CT scans are now routinely used to substantiate findings.

— **Indications for surgery** include (1) prevention of further nerve damage and deficits, (2) severe back and leg pain that does not respond sufficiently to an adequate course of conservative treatment (bed rest, traction, physical therapy, analgesia, back care exercises), and (3) a patient's optimistic expectation of the surgery's successful outcome with a positive mental attitude about rehabilitation and return to healthy behaviors. Positive clinical findings must be present. Emergency surgery is necessary for a totally extruded disc that is causing sensory and motor deficits in the lower extremities as well as a loss of bowel and bladder function (cauda equina syndrome).

— Whether or not **a spinal fusion** will be done following discectomy depends upon surgeon's skill, experience, and recommendations. Formerly advocated for chronic back victims, considerable controversy exists as to the value of a tradeoff of less pain for more disability. There is also a higher incidence of complications, in part because the surgery is longer, more complex, and involves greater exposure of tissues and bleeding. Rehabilitation is slower (four to five months in length) than with a simple first time discectomy/laminectomy (two to three months) that is performed for appropriate signs and symptoms in less than six weeks from onset of disc pathology.

— **Success of surgery** depends on (1) accuracy of diagnosis, extent and duration of disc pathology; (2) pre-op health (mental and physical) status of patient; and (3) excellence of surgery, recovery, and rehabilitation care. Success rates range from 50% to 90%. They are higher for athletes, airline pilots, and those with the energy, resiliency, and enthusiasm to overcome their disability; success rates are lower for middle class laborers, those with pending litigation or workers' compensation cases, those with previous back surgery, and those with emotional disturbances and negative mental attitudes.

— **Nursing responsibilities** include pre-op patient and family preparation (assessment, care, teaching), assistance with diagnostic tests; post-op care (prevention of complications, control of pain) and rehabilitation (patient/family education and discharge planning).

Specific Considerations, Potential Patient Outcomes, and Nursing Actions:

1) Pre-op
   Preparation

The patient will indicate s/he understands the nature of disc pathology, proposed surgery, and rehabilitation regimen; the patient will be physiologically and psychologically stabilized and prepared for surgery; the patient will express an optimistic, realistic, and reasonable expectation of a successful surgical outcome along with a positive attitude about own responsibility to participate in a return to healthy behavior:

— assess level of pt./family knowledge re: diagnosis, diagnostic tests, proposed surgery & rehabilitation plan; review, explain, & supplement needed info; explain diagnostic & surgical procedures carefully & honestly; use diagrams PRN;

— obtain informed, written consents for diagnostic tests, anesthesia, & operation;

— support & reinforce pt.'s optimism re: successful surgery; report to surgeon any pt. fears, doubts, negativism;

— explain importance & demonstrate with pt. post-op positioning, log-roll turning, body alignment, coughing, deep-breathing, passive & active leg exercises;

— if spinal fusion is to be done, a turning frame may be used or temporary plaster jacket; show these or pictures of them to pt., explaining & answering questions PRN; tell pt. about incision needed for bone graft & Hemovac that may be in place;

— obtain pre-op neurological check signs for post-op comparison; note all signs & symptoms, gait, mobility, altered bowel or bladder function, rashes or alterations in skin color & temp; take baseline vital signs including weight;

— refer to NCPG #2:44, "General Pre-Op Care," for additional nursing actions.

2) Rest and Exercise

The patient will maintain the prescribed postoperative position for functional healing of the spine; the patient will participate in gradual exercise and ambulation regimen, correctly turning, sitting, standing, and walking:

— prepare orthopedic post-op bed (or turning frame) according to hospital procedure;

— know & follow surgeon's specific orders for this pt.'s positioning, head elevation, turning, sitting, exercises, & ambulation program; review these with all potential care givers & be certain that nursing care plan is clearly written & specific;

— unless otherwise ordered, keep head of bed flat for 1st 12 hours post-op, then elevate it up to 30° PRN for comfort or feeding;

— have bedside commode available unless bathroom is close to pt.'s bed;

— turn pt. via log-roll method Q2H; support back & legs with pillows;

— check vital signs before & after moving pt. to sitting or standing positions; allow time for pt. to become accustomed to new position before progressing;

— unless otherwise ordered, assist pt. to sit on side of bed with legs dangling, approximately 4–6 hours following return from post-anesthesia recovery room; have pt. breathe deeply & assist to cough while supporting back & abdomen;

— upon written order, pt. may be helped to stand, then to walk about room on the 1st post-op day (unless a spinal fusion requiring longer period of immobility has been performed); progressively ambulate according to pt. tolerance & surgeon's orders;

— teach pt. that standing is less stressful on back than sitting, walking less than standing still;

— teach pt. back care principles (see NCPG # 3:41) & reinforce practice of back exercises as prescribed by physician or physical therapist; refer to NCPG # 3:42, "Back Exercises," PRN.

3) Prevention of Complications

The patient will be free of preventable complications or has them properly managed and promptly controlled; the patient will maintain effective normal body functions:

— refer to applicable nursing actions in NCPGs #2:41–43, "General Post-op Care, Part A: Support of Pulmonary Functions; Part B, Support of Cardiovascular Functions; and Part C, Support of Auxiliary Functions;"

— observe for signs & symptoms of complications specific to this surgery:

a) *thrombus*

• know that prolonged bed rest increases incidence of complications & rapid mobilization reduces incidence; know that current postsurgical programs encourage a far more rapid mobilization rate than in former years; know that most pts. (except those with spinal fusions) will be walking 1st or 2nd day post-op & gentle passive & active exercises will then be started by nurses or physical therapists;

• avoid pressure of pillows & pads under knees & calves of legs;

• keep elastic bandages or anti-embolic stockings in place as ordered, removing for 1 hour Q8H shift;

• have pt. flex toes, feet, ankles, & legs Q1H;

• observe legs & calves for inflammation, edema, pain/tenderness; measure & record size of calf & report increases of ½" or more;

• observe & report STAT chest pain, SOB, frothy or pink sputum, abnormal sudden change in vital signs, mental confusion; begin emergency O_2 at 4–6 liters/minute;

b) *neurological damage*

• perform neurological check on arms & legs Q30 minutes x 4, then Q1H x 8, then Q2H x 24 hours, then as deemed advisable; refer to NCPG #2:50 "Traction," for neurological check list of assessments;

• check pinprick sensations in all extremities Q2H;

• check ability to move arms & legs, fingers & toes at will;

• check for perianal sensation, rectal & bladder sphincter control Q2H;

c) *spinal fluid leakage*

• record & report all headaches; ask pt. to report onset of headache; know that headaches *may* mean leaking spinal fluid;

- observe dressing for clear spinal fluid drainage & report STAT; in interim, force fluids, keep head of bed flat, provide all physical care, keeping pt. on absolute bed rest;

d) *ileus*

- check abdomen for softness, for distention, for sounds Q2H; note expulsion of flatus & record;
- get order for rectal tube or low enema PRN for abdominal distention;

e) *infection and/or inflammation*

- record & report vital signs Q4H for at least 5 days post-op; know that pt. may be expected to have a temp of 100°F (37.8°–38.3°C) for 1st 72 hours post-op; report fevers of higher degrees or longer duration;
- report recurring or persisting pain at operative site;
- tell pt. to report severe muscle spasms to MD after discharge, as disc space infections usually occur 1–8 weeks postoperatively;
- note & report dressing drainage & odor, delayed healing, and/or inflammation of wound site;
- give scrupulous wound care & sterile dressing changes;
- report elevated eosinophil sedimentation rates to MD;
- give antibiotics carefully as ordered, therapeutically or prophylactically.

3) Pain Control   The patient will be free of pain and muscle spasm in the operative area or as comfortable as can be expected for the post-op day and status:
- provide sheet blankets, bed jackets, foot socks, & environmental controls for pt. comfort PRN;
- give pain medication prescribed but on a need-contingent (not a time-contingent) basis;
- utilize visual imagery, self-hypnosis, relaxation methods, & other pain management techniques to help pt. develop new skills for pain control; recognize & praise attempts to participate in ambulation, physical therapy, diversion, & positive thinking.

4) Fluids and Electrolytes   The patient will achieve fluid and electrolyte balance; the patient will progress to a regular nutritious diet; the patient will resume normal bowel and bladder elimination:
- provide ice chips & clear liquids as ordered, advancing to full liquids on 1st post-op day as tolerated;
- measure & record intake & output for at least 3 days, unless otherwise ordered;
- listen to abdomen & record return of bowel sounds;

— check voiding Q4H, reporting bladder distention & inability to void; obtain written order to allow male pts. to stand to void, before attempting to catheterize;

— give stool softeners as ordered; assist pt. to bedside commode for 1st post-op bowel movement; remain with pt. for safety precautions;

— advance pt. to full diet as tolerated.

5) Patient/ Family Education

The patient/family will verbalize an understanding of appropriate back care measures, back exercises and discharge instructions; the patient will demonstrate correct posture, body mechanics, and prescribed back exercises:

— provide pt. & family with written instructions re: care of operative site, back care regimen, & back exercises;

— demonstrate correct application & care of back brace, if one provided for this pt.;

— help pt. to list questions for MD re: restrictions & time table for resumption of driving, sexual intercourse, sports, housework, or job responsibilities; extent of surgery & health status of pts. vary, so answers must be tailored to individual.

Discharge Planning and Teaching Objectives/Outcomes

1) (Patient/Family/Significant Other) Can state restrictions re: activity, wound site, and return to driving, sports, or job.

2) Has a written set of back care measures and exercises; can demonstrate correct understanding and performance of them.

3) States s/he knows medications, dosage, indications, and side effects to be reported.

4) Knows to report promptly signs of illness, fever, increasing back pain or muscle spasms; has a follow-up medical appointment for rehabilitation regimen.

Recommended References

"Back Care." *NCP Guide #3:41*, 2nd Ed., Nurseco, 1983.

"Back Exercises." *NCP Guide #3:42*, 2nd Ed., Nurseco, 1983.

"Caring for the Laminectomy Patient: How to Strengthen Your Support," by J. Farrell. *Nursing 78*, May 1978:65–69.

"General Post-Op Care, Parts A, B, and C." *NCP Guides #2:41, 42, & 43*, 2nd Ed., Nurseco, 1980.

"General Pre-Op Care." *NCP Guide #2:44*, 2nd Ed., Nurseco, 1980.

"New Surgical Approach Minimizes Post-Op Pain," by E. Mulford. *RN*, February 1981:48–49.

"Nursing Care of the Patient with Recurrent Back Pain after Discectomy," by B. Sharp. *Journal of Neurosurgical Nursing*, April 1981:77–82.

"Surgery and Postsurgical Management of the Patient with Low Back Pain," by V. Mooney. *Physical Therapy*, August 1979:1000–1006.

"Traction: General Principles." *NCP Guide #2:50*, 2nd Ed., Nurseco, 1980.

The Patient with Low Back Pain

Definition: A perception of discomfort in the lumbar and/or sacral area of the spine or surrounding tissues; see below for specific definition.

LONG TERM GOAL: The patient will return to former roles and productive lifestyle, accommodating activities to current health status and back condition; the patient will understand the causes of own particular back pain and will be able to minimize recurrences through appropriate, recommended back care measures.

General Considerations:

— **Incidence and occurrence:** more than 75 million Americans have back problems; there are seven million new cases each year. Victims of low back pain are the second largest group of patients seeking care from family physicians; they make up one-third of all out-patient visits to orthopedic clinics. Low back pain is one of the largest single causes of worker absenteeism, with an estimated 93 million lost workdays annually. Low back pain occurs in both males and females of all classes and professions. While it affects young and old, the highest frequency is for the age group of 35–55 years of age. There is a higher than average risk in the tall and the obese.

— **Signs and symptoms:** high levels of physical and psychic tension accompanied by paralumbar muscle spasm and deep aching or sharp local pain. Overuse or misuse of back muscles → (leads to) muscle fatigue and strain → muscle spasm and contraction → reduced blood supply (ischemia) → pain → increased muscle spasm/ contraction and splinting of painful part → more ischemia → more pain. Tissue congestion and a loss of function/motion accompany pain.

— **Definitions:**
  - *strain*: a "pulled" or "overstretched" muscle, ligament, or tendon.
  - *sprain*: a more severe injury involving a "tearing" of a ligament, tendon, or muscle accompanied by tissue congestion with blood and fluid, and more immediate, severe, long-lasting, and widespread pain.
  - *sciatica*: sharp, shooting pain running down back of thigh and leg; associated with compression, inflammation, or trauma of sciatic nerve.
  - *facet joint dysfunction or facet arthralgia*: now used to describe the sudden "catch" in the back characterized by pain referred from the small vertebral facet joints down the leg to the knee or ankle and by a loss of back flexion and extension range of motion.

- *lordosis*: swayback with protruding abdominal muscles; connective tissues in back are shortened while abdominal tissues are stretched, producing abnormal curvature.
- *scoliosis*: an abnormal "S" shaped curvature of the spine involving unequal pull on back muscles, bones, and joints of the spine.
- *compression fracture*: a crushing together of a vertebral body, often associated with local soft tissue damage producing pain.
- *intervertebral disc*: consists of a nucleus of gelatinous pulp ("nucleus pulposus") surrounded by a fibrocartilage called fibrous annulus; the disc is the shock-absorbing cushion that lies between the cartilaginous end plates of each vertebra.
- *degenerative disc disease*: loss of normal spring-like turgor of the disc due to cellular changes in the fibrous annulus and dessication (dehydration) of the gelatinous nucleus; x-rays show narrowed interspaces and irregular cartilaginous edges; low back pain secondary to degenerative disc disease is increased by activity and subsides with bed rest; long periods of standing or sitting aggravate problem.
- *herniated, prolapsed, or "slipped" disc*: a protrusion of the nucleus through a ruptured annulus causing pressure on adjacent nerve roots, which produces lumbosacral and sciatic pain.
— **Causes:**
  - poor posture
  - obesity and/or pregnancy placing additional strain on weakened abdominal and back muscles
  - improper body mechanics (lifting, bending, twisting, pushing, etc.)
  - immobility and disuse of back, related to prolonged bed rest, sitting, or standing with lack of ambulation and appropriate exercise
  - congenital and developmental malformations (improper fusion of vertebrae, spina bifida, unequal leg length, etc.)
  - lumbar facet joint dysfunction syndrome
  - degenerative disease processes (osteo- and rheumatoid arthritis, osteoporosis, degenerative disc disease, etc.)
  - malignancies (primary or secondary tumors, metastases of spinal column)
  - trauma (strains, sprains, vertebral fractures, herniated nucleus pulposus, etc.)
  - iatrogenic (complications of one or more back surgeries, scar tissue formations, physician diagnostic and treatment errors)
  - psychologic or psychogenic (stress, worry, negative mental attitude, response to grief, boredom, repressed anger, etc.)
— **Diagnosis** is based on a complete history, physical, laboratory, and x-ray examination.

— **Treatment** aims to reduce pain; to identify and remove cause of pain; to prevent or minimize recurrence of low back pain; to resolve functional and behavioral factors related to pain experience and disability. A treatment regimen must be tailored to the individual's back problem, but usually includes more than one of the following components:

- *physical therapy*: including at least one or more of the following: improvement of posture and body mechanics, exercise program, moist heat, massage, ultrasound, gravity traction, electromyelographic biofeedback training, progressive relaxation therapy, surgical diathermy or facet denervation, spinal manipulation therapy (SMT), lumbosacral supports (elastic, velcro, or removable plaster body jackets); kinesiology;
- *psychological therapy*: testing, retraining, and rehabilitation for disabled self images, fears of disability and inability to return to former work (or any productive work); individual, group, and family counseling; occupational therapy; social services referral; behavioral modification therapy; pain control skills; crisis intervention and stress control skills; visual imagery and self-hypnosis techniques;
- *drug therapy*: appropriate individualized schedules of selected analgesics, anti-inflammatory agents, muscle relaxants, and tranquilizers followed by a gradual reduction to elimination of addicting medications;
- *surgical therapy*: standard laminectomy with macrodiscectomy; microdiscectomy; spinal fusion; chymopapain injections (done in Canada and at Johns Hopkins, Baltimore); implantation of dorsal column stimulators for transcutaneous nerve stimulation to control pain; trigger point injections with anesthetics and steroids; acupuncture.

— **Nursing responsibilities** include history, physical and mental assessment; assistance with diagnostic tests and treatment modalities, evaluation of the patient's response to treatment; and provision of education and counseling needed by patient and family to prevent and control recurrences of back pain.

Specific Considerations, Potential Patient Outcomes, and Nursing Actions:

1) Nursing   The patient's history and physical findings will be revealed; some causes of pain will be identified or ruled out; the
   Assessment patient's level and extent of back pathology and pain will be determined; the extent and level of disruption of impairment of the patient's physical and emotional function will be determined:

- — know that the most reliable & valid assessments are obtained by knowledgeable & experienced nurses who are qualified to do these; obtain training & supervision PRN;
- — complete nursing history form supplied by your agency (hospital, orthopedic clinic, pain clinic, or industrial setting); if none available, develop your own;

- observe & note pt.'s behavior, voice, & manner when s/he walks, sits, moves: note degree of flexion of neck, back, & legs;
- check pt. for scoliosis & lordosis;
- check passive & active range of motion & muscle strength;
- test plantar & dorsiflexion of ankles with opposing force;
- check foot inversion & eversion;
- test leg abduction bilaterally & unilaterally with opposition;
- measure pt.'s leg length (either have pt. lie prone with legs bent at knees, then measure from table surface to heel, *or* measure from medial malleoli to umbilicus or xiphoid process);
- measure circumference of legs at mid-calf & mid-thigh;
- with pt. in prone position, check hip extension with & without opposition;
- with pt. standing, check flexion forward, extension backwards & sidewards;
- evaluate symptoms of psychogenic origin by having pt. perform different variations of the same test;
- recheck ankle dorsiflexion by asking pt. to balance on each foot, raise up on toes, then walk on tip toes;
- recheck plantar flexion by asking pt. to walk on heels;
- recheck hip flexion by having pt. raise straight legs to 90° while supine and while sitting in a chair; know that reactions of pain show involvement of lumbar nerve roots;
- perform sensation tests to see which dermatomes (areas of skin) are affected; especially note reactions in skin areas innervated by suspected nerve root involved;
- complete all routine supplementary physical assessments, e.g., inspections, palpations, percussions, & auscultations;
- take careful nursing history covering both routine questions as well as those questions describing pain, impending legal actions or workers' compensation claims, psychosocial & family relationship factors, & suspected emotional disabilities.

2) Rest and Activity

The patient has reduced muscle spasm, muscle fatigue, and tension; the patient's pain is reduced; the patient's injured back tissues show gradual healing:
- prepare bed with a firm mattress & full-length bed board; utilize a foam pad, sheepskin, or flotation pad to provide more pt. comfort & to protect bony prominences from undue pressure; consider an overhead frame with trapeze to assist pt. in getting out of bed or turning;

— teach pt. how to flex spine in side-lying or supine positions with knees & hips flexed; teach pt. correct way to get into & out of bed;

— use pillow supports & folded towels to maintain correct body alignment (legs elevated, knees bent, head & shoulders slightly elevated, spine without lateral curvature but flexed);

— have pt. avoid prone & swayback positions;

— provide deep breathing, range of motion & muscle setting exercises for pt. on bed rest for more than 2 days;

— interpret to pt./family activity restrictions (up for elimination & shower only or whatever); provide basic comforts & necessary items within easy reach to avoid twisting, straining movements;

— if traction is ordered, prepare equipment & weights specified by MD; refer to NCPG #3:50, "Traction: General Principles."

3) Physical Therapy   The patient will experience relief of muscle spasm and reduced pain; the patient will develop stronger back, thigh, leg, and abdominal muscles; the patient will learn correct back care and back exercises:

— consult with physical therapist re: this pt.'s back problem & therapeutic program; review with pt. NCPGs #3:41, "Back Care," & #3:42, "Back Exercises," or their dept.'s pt. instruction forms to determine what parts meet this pt.'s needs; observe PT with pt. to learn how nursing staff can assist pt. between therapy sessions;

— assess pt.'s response to PT (level of understanding, application of new learning, practice of new skills, acceptance of regimen, degree of pain & spasm relief, etc.); reinforce, interpret, repeat explanations PRN; give pt. warm bath or shower & muscle relaxant meds PRN before exercise sessions;

— assist pt. to apply & wear abdominal & back supports correctly; provide skin care before & after wear; observe & treat minor skin irritations;

— meet with PT on follow-up basis to discuss evaluation of pt.'s response to physical therapy; review goals & revise therapeutic plan accordingly.

4) Pain Control   The patient will experience and report diminished pain/discomfort; the patient will require fewer and milder medications for pain control; the patient will experience less muscle spasm, emotional tension, anxiety, and reactive depression associated with pain; the patient will exhibit less pain-centered behavior, habits, communications, and attitudes; the patient will demonstrate new skills for pain management and reduction that s/he can use at home and work; the patient will demonstrate increased activity, independence, and ability to cope with role responsibilities:

— discuss with pt. & family present back pain, previous experience with this type of pain, measures that have given relief, & pt.'s own perceptions & beliefs of how nursing can best help relieve this pain; assess pt.'s preadmission use of pain medication (types, frequency, dosage levels, how administered, related use of other drugs or chemicals);

— based on assessment of pt.'s problems, needs, & concerns, as well as consultation with MD & with pain specialist, devise a plan for pain management; involve the pt. & family; elicit their cooperation & participation in decisions;

— explore possibilities of spasm, tension, & pain reducers such as biofeedback training, transcendental meditation, relaxation techniques, visual imagery, self-hypnosis, yoga, acupuncture, color or music therapy, hydrotherapy, dorsal electrical stimulators, trigger-point injection treatments, behavior modification methods, individual or group psychological counseling, & occupational therapy;

— help pt. to accept pain as a perception rather than as a sensation; refer to NCPG #1:30, "The Patient Experiencing Pain;"

— obtain permission to try ice packs or warm, moist heat therapy for 15 minutes TID;

— give back rubs (gentle massage using heels of hands in long, slow strokes) ad lib & at least twice daily;

— give anti-inflammatory medications & muscle relaxants as ordered, but give analgesics & sedatives on a pain-contingent basis rather than a time-contingent basis; reward diminishing frequency of requests for pain relief; give bedtime meds with warm milk to promote sleep; observe & record response to meds;

— provide recognition & praise for healthy pain management behaviors such as ambulation, showing interest in people or activities other than self, participation in physical therapy or stress management exercises, & positive mental attitudes;

— refer PRN to psychologist/psychiatrist, minister, social worker, vocational rehabilitation technician, or clinical nurse specialist in pain management;

— recognize, identify, & control negative feelings & care behaviors of self or other nursing personnel toward pain-centered, dependent patient; open, frank admission & discussion of these negative attitudes can be very helpful in learning to control or reduce them.

5) Psycho-
social
Adjustment,
Patient and
Family
Education

The patient will progress from a pain-centered dependent, disabled self-image to a more active, independent, self-controlled person with increased ability to cope with role responsibilities; the patient will participate actively in discussions of personal problems, feelings, attitudes, and self-limiting behaviors; the patient will assist increasingly in defining own problems, setting goals, and making decisions:

— interview pt. & family to analyze job demands, home responsibilities, social service needs, & family role responsibilities; assess sources of physical & psychic stress along with effective or ineffective coping strategies; identify negative, non-productive, self-limiting habits, attitudes, beliefs, & feelings re: own disability & pain;

— after consultation with MD & other therapeutic team members, make appropriate referrals to social services, vocational rehabilitation or occupational therapist, psychologist/psychiatrist, community/school/occupational health nurse, & discharge coordinator; help coordinate mutual goal-directed joint team effort & cooperation for the patient's benefit;

— teach pt. & family anatomy of spine, correct body mechanics & posture, back exercises (NCPG #3:42) & principles of back care (NCPG #3:41);

— teach pt. & family techniques of progressive relaxation & more effective coping strategies of psychic stress management (NCPG #5:49);

— teach assertiveness skills & how to dialogue more effectively with self in order to control self-defeating self-criticism;

— openly confront & discuss with pt. attempts to delay rehabilitation process & progress by either minimal performance or over-zealous compliance with regimen; restate self-help goals & help to understand how s/he can undermine or reinforce treatment plan;

— recognize, reward, openly acknowledge, & praise pt. behavior changes toward a more productive, optimistic, independent lifestyle; encourage attempts to attain control over pain experience.

Discharge Planning and Teaching Objectives/Outcomes

1) (Patient/Family/Significant Other) Can state causes of own back pain and what s/he must do to prevent or control recurrence.
2) Has received and read copies of NCPGs #3:41, "Back Care," and #3:42, "Back Exercises," or other supplied patient instruction materials.
3) Demonstrates an understanding and acceptance of back care principles by using improved posture and body mechanics while standing, sitting, lying down, lifting, or performing activities.
4) Can demonstrate exercises correctly without assistance; indicates willingness to follow a regular program of exercise/rest and diet control.
5) Can identify medications, their purpose, side effects, dosage, and administration constraints.
6) Knows immediate first aid measures for handling a recurrence of sudden back pain.

Recommended References

"An Innovative Program for the Restoration of Patients with Chronic Back Pain," by H. Gottlieb et al. *Physical Therapy*, August 1979:996-999.
"An Occupational Therapy Program for Chronic Back Pain," by A. Flower et al. *American Journal of Occupational Therapy*, April 1981:243-248.
"Back Care." *NCP Guide #3:41*, 2nd Ed., Nurseco, 1983.
"Back Exercises." *NCP Guide #3:42*, 2nd Ed., Nurseco, 1983.
'Degenerative Disease or 'Slipped' Disc?" by E. Mulford. *RN*, February 1981:45-47.
How to Care for Your Back, by H. Keim. Englewood Cliffs, NJ: Prentice-Hall, 1981.
"Low Back Pain," by J. Pace. *Critical Care Update*, February 1980:8-9.
"Nursing Assessment of a Patient with Low Back Pain," by M. Hitch. *The Orthopedic Nurses Association Journal*, December 1979:484-488.
"Nursing Care of the Patient with Recurrent Back Pain after Discectomy," by B. Sharp. *Journal of Neurosurgical Nursing*, April 1981:77-82.
"The Patient Experiencing Pain." *NCP Guide #1:30*, 2nd Ed., Nurseco, 1980.
"Stress Management." *NCP Guide #5:49*, Nurseco, 1981.
"That Aching Back!" *Time*, July 14, 1980:30-38.
"Traction: General Principles." *NCP Guide #2:50*, 2nd Ed., Nurseco, 1980.

The Patient with a Herniated Intervertebral Disc: Medical Management

Definition: An intervertebral disc (or disk) consists of a nucleus of gelatinous pulp ("nucleus pulposus") surrounded by a fibrocartilage called annulus fibrosis; the disc is the flat, round, shock-absorbing cushion that lies between the cartilaginous end plates of each vertebra. A protrusion of the nucleus through a ruptured annulus causes pressure on adjacent nerve roots, producing lumbosacral and sciatic pain extending down the leg. This extruded nucleus is also called a herniated nucleus pulposus (HNP). A bulging of a weakened disc through the end plates without a torn annulus is commonly known as a "slipped" or prolapsed disc.

LONG TERM GOAL: The patient will return to former roles and productive lifestyle, accommodating activities to current health status and back condition; the patient participates in a long-term back care regimen designed to prevent recurrences of back pain.

General Considerations:

— **Incidence and occurrence:** disc herniations are more frequent in men and are associated with insufficient physical exercise as well as with participation in certain sports (golf, bowling, and baseball, which involve bending and torsion stresses most likely to produce trauma). Two top risk factors are sedentary occupations and driving a motor vehicle; the intradiscal pressure is distinctly and significantly higher in the sitting position than in the standing position.

— **Cause** of herniation is believed to be increased intradiscal pressure against a weakened disc wall. Degenerative disc disease increases the load placed on the annulus. There is a loss of normal spring-like turgor of the disc due to cellular changes in the fibers and dehydration of the gelatinous nucleus; narrowed vertebral interspaces and irregular cartilaginous surfaces further diminish normal disc function. Aging, trauma, and poor disc nutrition (associated with inactivity, poor body mechanics, and stress factors) contribute to the speed of disc degeneration.

— **Signs and symptoms:** immediate and sudden loss of mobility accompanied by excruciating lower back pain extending down one or both legs.

— **Emergency care,** until seen by an MD, includes:
  - a back-lying position on a flat, firm surface with legs bent at hips and knees, with lower legs elevated on the seat of a chair or a stack of cushions at least 46 cm (18") high;
  - an ice pack beneath lumbar curve; and
  - 600 mg (10 gr) aspirin orally.

— **Diagnosis** is based on a complete history, physical, laboratory and x-ray examination.

— **Treatment** aims are to reduce pain; to identify and remove cause of pain due to pressure on spinal nerve roots; to prevent further loss of function; and to rehabilitate patient to former mobility status. Studies show that 85–90% of patients demonstrate remission of symptoms in less than two months on conservative treatment that includes bed rest (firm mattress on bed boards), lumbar traction, analgesics, anti-inflammatory agents and steroids, physical therapy, back exercises, back braces, and (sometimes) weight-reducing diets. For patients who have not sufficiently improved on the above medical regimen after eight weeks, and for those who have a positive and optimistic attitude about the benefits of an operation to relieve their back problem, surgery is often indicated. A macrodiscectomy and laminectomy with spinal fusion is commonly performed although a newer and simpler operation, a microdiscectomy, is sometimes done.

Chemonucleolysis, the nonoperative removal of displaced lumbar disc material by using the enzyme chymopapain, is being done in Canada and experimentally in Baltimore. It has been shown to be successful in up to 80% of carefully selected patients who have a herniation of a single disc and who have had no prior unsuccessful spinal surgery. Ambulation is quicker, hospital stays are shorter (four to five days), pain relief is dramatic, and the patient can often return to work in seven or eight weeks. Nevertheless, clinical trials continue under carefully supervised research methodology. Now approved for use in the US.

Injection of collagenase in the treatment of a herniated lumbar disc has also been used successfully in 20–60% of selected patients not helped by other methods of conservative treatment.

— **Nursing responsibilities** include nursing history, physical and mental assessment, assistance with diagnostic tests and treatment modalities, evaluation of the patient's response to treatment, and provision of education and counseling needed by patient and family to prevent and control further episodes of disc problems.

Specific Considerations, Potential Patient Outcomes, and Nursing Actions:

1) Nursing Assessment	The patient's history and physical findings will be revealed; causes of back pain other than disc extrusion will be ruled out; the extent and level of back pathology, pain, and impairment of function will be determined:

— refer to NCPG #3:09, "The Patient with Low Back Pain;"

— know that discogenic pain is usually intermittent, becoming more frequent & severe depending on the degree of herniation, the amount & direction of disc extrusion, & the performance of certain maneuvers or movements; know that pt. may experience both lumbar & sciatic pain simultaneously or separately; know that the pt.'s history of pain is likely to be related either to a single traumatic event or to awakening from a night's sleep with sciatic pain extending into buttock & down one or both extremities; usually the lumbar pain gradually worsens over days or weeks followed by intense, disabling sciatic pain that sends pt. quickly to MD; know that, typically, discogenic pain is worsened by anterior & lateral flexion of the spine as well as by rotational movements, by laughing, sneezing, coughing, or straining at defecation, by raising the straight leg to 80 or 90° while pt. is supine, & by compressing jugular veins (Naffziger test);

— note any pt. attempts to relieve nerve root pressure by leaning toward affected side or flexing affected leg at knee;

— feel for muscle spasm & tautness at the L4-L5 & L5-S1 levels where most lumbar disc lesions occur;

— note any numbness, weakness, paralysis, or decreased reflexes along affected nerve pathway of leg, ankle, & foot.

For 2) Rest and Activity, 3) Physical Therapy, 4) Pain Control, and 5) Psychosocial Adjustment and Patient and Family Education, see these considerations in NCPG #3:09, "The Patient with Low Back Pain."

Discharge Planning and Teaching Objectives/Outcomes
See NCP Guide #3:09, "The Patient with Low Back Pain."

Recommended References
"Acute Symptomatic Disk Prolapse," by R. Kessler. *Physical Therapy*, August 1979:978-987.
"Back Care." *NCP Guide #3:41*, 2nd Ed., Nurseco, 1983.
"Back Exercises." *NCP Guide #3:42*, 2nd Ed., Nurseco, 1983.
"Biomechanics of the Lumbar Intervertebral Disk: A Review," by G. Jensen. *Physical Therapy*, June 1980:765-773.
"Degenerative Disease or 'Slipped' Disc?" by E. Mulford. *RN*, February 1981:45-47.
"Injections for Ruptured Spinal Discs: Chemonucleolysis," by M. Schneider. *Aches & Pains*, October 1981:20-23.
"Nursing Assessment of a Patient with Low Back Pain," by M. Hitch. *The Orthopedic Nurses Association Journal*, December 1979:484-489.
"The Patient Experiencing Pain." *NCP Guide #1:30*, 2nd Ed., Nurseco, 1980.
"The Patient with Lower Back Pain." *NCP Guide #3:09*, 2nd Ed., Nurseco, 1983.
"Stress Management." *NCP Guide #5:49*, Nurseco, 1981.
"Traction: General Principles." *NCP Guide #2:50*, 2nd Ed., Nurseco, 1980.

The Patient with Osteoarthritis

Definition: Osteoarthritis is a degenerative bone and joint disease involving pitting, disintegration, and loss of elasticity in cartilage surfaces between bones.

LONG TERM GOAL: The patient will attain the optimal level of functioning within the physical limitations of osteoarthritis; s/he will perform activities of daily living within a prescribed treatment regimen, demonstrating a realistic knowledge of the disease and its treatment.

General Considerations:

— **Occurrence:** increases with advancing age (in those over 60, x-ray signs are evident in 97%); twice as common in females as males.

— **Types:** *primary* type affects women in their forties and fifties; underlying factors include heredity and hormonal changes; commonly involves swollen end joints of fingers and toes (Heberden's nodes), which can sometimes be quite painful. *Secondary* type affects most men and women over 65; underlying factors include obesity, poor posture, and minor injuries; commonly involves knees, hips, and spine.

— **Symptoms:** joint pain, either aching soreness or constant, nagging-type, progressive during day with fatigue and usage; pain alleviated with rest, although that causes temporary stiffness and limitation of joint motion. Symptoms are exacerbated by weather (cold and dampness), stress, obesity, poor posture, minor injuries, and overusage *or* inactivity of joints.

— **Treatment** aims to control pain and improve joint function; regimen commonly includes antiarthritic drugs, a balanced diet, optimum combinations of rest and exercise, and patient/family/significant other (SO) education appropriate to needs. Supportive and assistive devices are sometimes indicated and corrective orthopedic surgery of the most seriously affected joints is currently advocated.

— **Nursing responsibilities** include assessment of patient/family/SO's knowledge/attitudes/abilities and limitations relevant to osteoarthritis condition; provision of nursing care in activities of daily living (ADL) and range of motion (ROM) exercises; implementation of prescribed therapeutic regimen; counseling and teaching as necessary; and coordination of continuing care or services.

Specific Considerations, Potential Patient Outcomes, and Nursing Actions:

1) Medication   The patient will experience reduced pain and fibrositis:
   — administer aspirin & other analgesics liberally as ordered; observe & record tolerance, results, side effects;
   — if corticosteroids are given during acute episodes, observe carefully pt.'s reactions, daily I&O, BP, weight, vital signs; refer to NCPG #5:43, "Drugs: Corticosteroids."

2) Rest and Activity   The patient will maintain functional position and optimum joint mobility; the patient will experience reduced muscle strain and weakness; the patient will be free of flexion deformities:
   — during painful exacerbation phase, provide sufficient rest with joints in functional alignment; when pain is controlled, provide appropriate exercises (as selected by PT, MD, or orthopedic nurse) PRN for improved muscle strength, tone, & mobility (not endurance);
   — perform ROM exercises 1–2 x daily; see NCPG #1:47, "Range of Motion Exercises;"
   — practice with pt. for better understanding & performance between PT sessions;
   — keep muscles & joints reasonably warm before & after activity using bed socks, pajama bottoms, heating pads, blankets, etc; provide gradual "cool down" process to avoid muscle stiffening & pt. chilling;
   — identify, teach, & reinforce measures that promote good posture, correct joint function, maintain body alignment, eliminate fatigue & strain; stress importance of letting others lift or carry heavy loads;
   — assess & discuss with pt. his/her physical limitations & need for safety/assistive devices, e.g., grab bars in toilet, tub, & shower, straight-back chairs, light-weight cooking utensils, canes or braces, etc.;
   — refer to NCPG #2:32, "Aged Patient: Exercises for Patients Over 65," PRN.

3) Diet   The patient will ingest a well-balanced diet of optimal nutrition for ideal body weight range:
   — consult with pt. & family for likes, dislikes, allergies, cultural & age-related food preferences/practices, appetite, & eating patterns;
   — identify other medical problem-related dietary requirements;
   — explain, explore, & support need for reducing caloric intake in overweight pts.; refer to NCPG #5:41, "Diet: Weight Control;"
   — observe & record acceptance of meals on diet; health teach pt./family PRN.

4) Psycho- logical Adjustment and Rehabil- itation	The patient will adjust adaptively to chronic diagnosis and will achieve an active, cooperative acceptance of thera- peutic regimen and home care program:

The patient will adjust adaptively to chronic diagnosis and will achieve an active, cooperative acceptance of therapeutic regimen and home care program:

— ask pt. to share experiences with pain, & listen for cues & clues to alleviation; encourage faith in MD & use power of suggestion or distraction in association with administration of analgesics; see NCPG #1:30, "The Patient Experiencing Pain;"

— discuss & clarify beliefs & knowledge of osteoarthritis (dangers of delaying treatment, quackery & misconceptions re: effectiveness of diet, climate, copper bracelets, "buckeye" or chestnut seed in pocket, etc.);

— know that emotional upsets & tension make condition worse; share this with pt.; attempt to determine & to alleviate causes of stress; help pt. cope with stress more effectively & discuss with pt. new or alternative methods to try; refer to NCPG #5:49, "Stress Management;"

— assist pt. to perform basic ADL using assistive devices PRN correctly; see NCPGs #1:49, "Teaching Patients: General Suggestions," & #1:50, "Specific Plan for Skills & Procedures;"

— if surgery (joint fusion, artificial joints, bone resections, etc.) is advocated, explore pt.'s feelings about surgery, possible outcome, family adjustments, etc.; support realistic decisions;

— assess need for vocational rehabilitation, convalescent hospital, or home health care assistance; consult with MD & social worker re: referrals desired;

— obtain family's understanding, acceptance, & assistance in all aspects of patient care planning, implementation, & evaluation.

Discharge Planning and Teaching Objectives/Outcomes

1) (Patient/Family/Significant Other) Can explain in own words basic facts about osteoarthritis (e.g., nature of disease, symptoms, aggravating factors, effects of treatment to control pain and to prevent disability).

2) Has received, read, and discussed The Arthritis Foundation pamphlet supplied by medical personnel ("So You Have . . . Arthritis").

3) Has identified purpose, actions, side effects, prescribed dosage, and PRN conditions for each medication prescribed.

4) Can correctly demonstrate range of motion and other prescribed exercises for home usage, correct posture and body mechanics; verbalizes acceptance of physical limitations and a willingness to plan activities accordingly, minimizing fatigue and stress.

5) Has been provided with a written set of instructions re: activities, exercise, medications, use of self-help devices, and appointment for medical follow-up; has verbalized confidence and willingness to carry out recommendations.

6) Has been evaluated for assistance (financial, vocational, convalescent hospital or home health care) and appropriate referrals have been made to state and local agencies.

7) Has received information re: additional community resources and services; has at least one community health source person's name and number, besides doctor, in order to get help and information.

Recommended References

"Aged Patient: Exercises for Patients Over 65." *NCP Guide #2:32*, 2nd Ed., Nurseco, 1980.

"Diet: Weight Control." *NCP Guide #5:41*, Nurseco, 1981.

"Drugs: Corticosteroids." *NCP Guide #5:43*, Nurseco, 1981.

"If Your Patient's Joints Hurt, the Reason May be Osteoarthritis," by M. Nowotny. *Nursing 80*, September 1980:39–41.

"Range of Motion Exercises." *NCP Guide #1:47*, 2nd Ed., Nurseco, 1980.

So You Have . . . Arthritis (Patient Handbook Series). Atlanta, GA.: Arthritis Foundation (3400 Peachtree Road NE, 30326).

"Stress Management." *NCP Guide #5:49*, Nurseco, 1981.

"Teaching Patients: General Suggestions." *NCP Guide #1:49*, 2nd Ed., Nurseco, 1980.

"Teaching Patients: Specific Plan for Skills and Procedures." *NCP Guide #1:50*, 2nd Ed., Nurseco, 1980.

"The Patient Experiencing Pain." *NCP Guide #1:30*, 2nd Ed., Nurseco, 1980.

The Patient with Osteoporosis

Definition: Osteoporosis is a bone disorder characterized by a loss of bone minerals, a slowing of bone formation, and a brittleness or loss of bone density.

LONG TERM GOAL: The patient will return to optimal activity and nutritive state, averting further bone destruction and reducing incidence of complications.

General Considerations

— **Occurrence:** increases with age, more common in those over 50; especially seen in white women of northern European descent; seen commonly in Oriental women but not often in blacks, who have greater mineral density at all ages; associated with sedentary inactivity; thin women at greater risk than obese women, who may have a higher endogenous estrogen production.

— **Types:** *primary* (formerly known as "post-menopausal" or "senile") osteoporosis is a true disease related to a combination of factors (inadequate calcium, dietary and non-dietary factors); *secondary* osteoporosis is caused by other diseases and/or their treatment (such as corticosteroid therapy).

— **Signs and symptoms:** pain (in legs or lumbar region related to compression fractures or to associated muscle spasm); shorter stature; dowager's hump; periodontal disease; susceptibility to fractures of weight-bearing joints (commonly wrist, hip, spine).

— **Diagnosis** is based on laboratory studies of serum calcium and hormone levels; morphometric analysis of biopsy material; and routine x-rays showing vertebral crush fractures (*note*: routine x-rays do not show a 10–20% loss of bone mass, only upwards of 30%; by that time other symptoms are apparent).

— **Treatment** aims are to alleviate symptoms and to avert further bone deterioration; the regimen includes:
  1) corrective diet of low fat, moderate protein, increased calcium in optimal ratio with phosphorus;
  2) mineral supplements of calcium, sodium, potassium, citric acid, and sometimes sodium fluoride (which has been shown experimentally to help stabilize bone tissue);
  3) adequate exposure to sunlight's ultraviolet rays or Vitamin D supplements to promote absorption of calcium (*note*: Vitamin D in excess amounts of 20,000 IUs daily causes hypercalcemia and increases bone resorption with risk of fracture);
  4) moderate exercise (weight-bearing type such as walking, riding a bicycle, or dancing) at least 30 minutes three times weekly to ensure continued stimulation of osteoblastic activity;

5) hormone therapy; estrogen is no longer approved by FDA for treatment of osteoporosis, but is still employed because of evidence it prevents age-related bone atrophy in post-menopausal women; decision to use must be based on a benefit-risk analysis for a specific patient. If used, patient must be watched for side effects of salt and water retention, increased blood pressure levels, breast fullness, & increased risk of endometrial cancer (unless hysterectomy has been performed); more frequent D&Cs with endometrial biopsies will be indicated. With regard to anabolic steroids, it is known that weak androgen sex hormones may not increase bone formation but do reduce the rate of bone resorption or dissolution, so are believed to be especially helpful with secondary osteoporosis induced by cortisone therapy.

— **Nursing responsibilities** include observation, assessment, intervention, and patient education re: patient's health habits and osteoporosis therapeutic regimen.

Specific Considerations, Potential Patient Outcomes, and Nursing Actions:

1) Diet   The patient will accept, ingest, and absorb a nutritionally-balanced diet necessary to promote bone formation:

— assess pt.'s dietary needs, cultural & personal preferences, mealtime environment, motivation for food preparation, knowledge of basic foods & nutrients, dentition, appetite, & relevant health problems;

— know that excess fat & protein decreases calcium absorption; know that excess phosphorus causes excess calcium loss from bones, so need to evaluate phosphate in diet via carbonated beverages, processed meats, & bakery products; know that 1980 RDA for calcium is 800 mg & for Vit. D is 200 IUs; teach pt. that this requirement can be met with 2 cups of low fat milk a day plus a variety of other foods; for the lactose-intolerant pt., substitute other foods plus calcium supplements;

— with dietician & pt.'s family or caretaker, plan a series of daily menus that include suitable amounts of milk, cheese, ice cream, poultry, fish, legumes, fresh fruits & vegetables (especially dark-green, leafy types); discuss plan with pt., making adjustments PRN;

— give vitamin & mineral supplements as prescribed by MD, explaining dangers of excessive intake; note lab reports for increased levels of calcium;

— observe, evaluate, & record pt.'s tolerance of diet; note & resolve problems.

2) Exercise
and
Physical
Activity

The patient will maintain or increase physical activity level recommended to prevent disuse atrophy and further bone destruction; the patient will maintain optimal muscle strength and joint mobility:
— refer to NCPGs #2:45, "Hazards of Immobility," #2:32, "Exercises for Patients Over 65," & #1:47, "ROM Exercises;"
— get pt. up at least BID for 10-minute walks with needed assistance to prevent falls; when tolerated, encourage longer walks & swimming, dancing, or bicycling (including a stationary, indoor type);
— urge moderate exposure to sunshine, explaining that ultraviolet rays on skin produce (endogenous) Vit. D needed for calcium absorption.

3) Safety
Precautions

The patient will remain free of preventable fractures and other incapacitating injuries:
— provide sufficient lighting in room, hallway, & bathroom; keep signal cord easily accessible;
— ensure that pt. has cane, walker, or personnel for walking assistance; have the pt. wear firm-soled shoes; avoid use of throw rugs in home environments; provide grip-bars in hallways, toilets, bathtub, & shower stalls;
— see that pt. has bedboard under mattress & full length bedrails in place while sleeping;
— if needed, arrange for back & leg braces or abdominal, wrist, knee, & ankle supports; know that back braces reduce mobility & weight-bearing muscular activity, so use only to ambulate previously bedridden pts.; consider substituting a girdle PRN & physical therapy to strengthen back muscles;
— caution pt. not to lift or carry much weight or bend over a great deal; teach pt. to avoid (if possible) fast, bumpy riding in autos or buses.

4) Hormone
Therapy

The patient will maintain hormone levels consistent with retardation of osteoporotic condition while minimizing or controlling undesirable side effects:
— administer hormones as ordered, observing & reporting pt.'s response;
— check & record daily weight & BP; report changes;
— discuss with MD & with pt. the desirable & undesirable effects of hormone therapy; encourage pt. to ask questions & express feelings;
— if on estrogen therapy, observe & record vaginal bleeding; arrange for periodic cancer-screening tests; be sure that pt. is performing monthly breast examinations correctly;
— if on androgen therapy, note facial hairiness, nausea, GI disturbances, signs of salt & water retention.

Discharge Planning and Teaching Objectives/Outcomes

1) (Patient/Family/Significant Other) Has received a written set of instructions re: diet, exercise, safety precautions and medications; has expressed confidence, understanding, and willingness to carry out instructions.

2) Has been evaluated for discharge assistance; has received appropriate referrals to local agencies; has information re: TLC (Transportation, Lunch, & Counseling), Meals-on-Wheels, other senior citizen services in own community.

Recommended References

"The Aged Patient: Exercises for Patients Over 65." *NCP Guide #2:32*, 2nd Ed., Nurseco, 1980.

"Dx: Osteoporosis, Rx: Patient Teaching," by E. Rausch and C. Haessig. *The Journal of Practical Nursing*, February 1981:26–27, 39.

"Hazards of Immobility." *NCP Guide #2:45*, 2nd Ed., Nurseco, 1980.

"Range of Motion Exercises." *NCP Guide #1:47*, 2nd Ed., Nurseco, 1980.

"Rational Management of Osteoporosis," by R. Marcus. *Hospital Formulary*, March 1981:265–281.

The Patient with Renal Failure: Acute

Definition: A sudden loss of renal function, frequently associated with another disease process, that is manifested by insufficient bladder urine. The result is a rise in the nitrogenous waste products and a hypervolemic state.

LONG TERM GOAL: The patient will be assisted to restore normal kidney function and to resume usual activities and roles.

General Considerations:
— **Categories** of acute renal failure (ARF):
  1) **pre-renal failure** (hypoperfused kidneys), associated with any process leading to a loss of blood volume → decreased cardiac output → decreased renal flow → renal ischemia and oliguria (urine volume less than 400 ml/24 hours). *Precipitating factors*: often caused by a drop in BP which results in dehydration due to salt and water loss from fluid deprivation, hemorrhage, GI losses, or burns. Other factors are sequestration ("third space") syndrome, septic shock, overdose of anti-hypertensive medication, congestive heart failure, myocardial infarction, hepato-renal syndrome, or major vascular surgery. Pre-renal failure refers to a decrease in circulation that occurs prior to the kidney failure itself.
  2) **intrarenal failure** (diseased kidneys), associated with prolonged and severe pre-renal failure that results in renal parenchymal injury and acute tubular necrosis. It is usually a result of a phenomenon that effects the kidney directly. May be caused by acute glomerulonephritis and pyelonephritis, transfusion reaction with massive hemolysis, disseminated intravascular coagulation (DIC), myoglobinuria, eclampsia, malignant hypertension, or renal artery/vein occlusion. *Precipitating factors* include nephrotoxic therapeutic agents (e.g., gentamycin, methicillin, Kanamycin, PAS, halothane, Amphotericin B), diagnostic or osmotic agents, organic solvents, heavy metals, chemicals (e.g., pesticides, mushrooms), and physical agents (e.g., radiation, electroshock).
  3) **post-renal failure** (obstructed kidneys), is caused by an obstruction of the collecting system as in calculi, prostatic hypertrophy, or tumors of prostate, pelvis, or bladder. Post-renal failure refers to decreased renal function resulting from a problem associated with the kidney structure beyond the pelvis of the kidney.
— **Common manifestations:** anuria, oliguria, anorexia, N&V, increased rate and depth of respirations, fluid retention (manifested by body edema), hypertension, bleeding tendencies, dry mucous membranes, itchy skin, urine odor on breath, CNS disturbances (lethargy, drowsiness, headache, muscle twitching, convulsions), and azotemia (accumulation of nitrogenous waste products in the blood with resultant increased levels of uric acid, creatinine, and BUN). Uremic frost (from excretion of waste products via the skin) is seen only in untreated terminal uremia.

— **Progress of disease:** oliguric period (may last twelve to fourteen days), followed by the diuretic phase (urinary output gradually increases to two to six liters/QD), then the convalescent and repair phase (may last six to twelve months).

— **Prognosis** is guarded (mortality rate in ARF is 50%), but the kidney has a remarkable ability to recover from insult. ARF is reversible if the disease process is recognized early and treatment started immediately. Of the patients that die from ARF, 95% can be attributed to sepsis.

— **Treatment** aims are (1) to diagnose and remove the cause(s) of renal failure and (2) to maintain the patient in as normal a state as possible in order to promote repair and restoration of renal tissue and function.

— **Dialysis** is utilized if response to conservative therapy is poor, in order to remove waste products and maintain the patient until renal recovery occurs. See NCPGs #3:03, "The Patient on Dialysis: Hemodialysis," and #3:05, "Peritoneal Dialysis." Indications for dialysis in ARF include irreversible metabolic acidosis, hyperkalemia, N&V, pulmonary edema, pericarditis, or GI bleeding.

— **Nursing responsibilities** include close observation and monitoring of the patient's fluid and electrolyte status, nutritional and psychological states; preparing the patient for dialysis (both physically and emotionally), and teaching patient/family/significant other (SO) about the disease process, prescribed therapeutic regimen, and prognosis.

Specific Considerations, Potential Patient Outcomes, and Nursing Actions:

1) Fluids and Electrolytes   The patient will accept fluid restrictions in order to maintain fluid and electrolyte balance; the patient will receive a fluid intake adjusted *only* to body need during the oliguric phase:

— record accurate fluid intake (IV, ultrasonic nebulization, oral, gastric feedings, lavage) & output (urine, feces, emesis, suction wound drainage) QH & then Q8H; pt. usually given amounts excreted + 500 ml daily (average insensible loss through skin & lungs);

— note & chart composition of body fluid losses;

— if pt. has an IV, regulate gtts/minute according to MD's orders;

— weigh QD, at same time with same clothing; use a bed scale PRN (weight gain should not occur unless excessive salt & water are administered;

— assess pt.'s hydration status by analysing weight changes (a gain or loss of 1 kg/2.2 lbs = a gain or loss of 1 liter of fluid), skin turgor, thirst, mucous membrane moisture, I&O, & edema;

— if urinary catheter used, ensure it is patent, unkinked, & secured to bed with tape &/or a pin, so that no tension is pulling on it; never leave catheter clamped unless you have a specific timed order from MD (see NCPG #2:39, "Catheters: Indwelling Urinary"); if pt. is anuric, remove catheter as ordered by MD;

— know normal levels of serum electrolytes, CBC, & blood gases; check lab. results & report to MD PRN;
— know, observe for, & chart signs & symptoms of electrolyte imbalance; report to MD; see NCPGs #3:48 & 49, "Fluids & Electrolytes;"
— be aware that hyperkalemia is life-threatening to ARF pts.; follow EKG & watch for peaked T waves.

2) Nutrition

The patient will accept controlled dietary restrictions in order to reduce amount of nitrogenous waste products in the blood; the patient will receive an adequate caloric intake that will minimize protein breakdown:
— provide a diet high in biological value protein (meat, eggs, fish, fowl—60–80 gm QD); give high caloric, essential amino acids supplement such as Ensure; if only calories are needed, use products such as Polycase & Hi-Cal;
— provide a diet *high in carbohydrates* (100 gms or more QD), low in potassium (see NCPG #2:48, "Potassium Imbalance"), & *low in sodium* (10 mEq/day); thirst will not be present if Na & water are properly managed (see NCPG #3:44, "Diet: Sodium-Restricted");
— maintain hyperalimentation catheter (this provides the basic essential amino acids in a high caloric solution in order to reduce the pt.'s tissue breakdown, therefore reducing azotemia); review NCPG #3:50, "Hyperalimentation;" when pt. is able to take oral intake, continue with Ensure.

3) Prevention of Complications

The patient will be free of preventable complications; the patient will maintain cardiovascular integrity:
— observe for, chart, & report to MD any signs or symptoms that may indicate complications; know that common ones, observations, & critical care include:
  • *pericarditis* with increasing effusion leading to tamponade, recognized by a paradoxical pulse & decreased pulse pressure; institute written medical procedure for emergency Rx of pericardial tamponade if one is available for your unit;
  • *acute hypertension*: give meds as ordered; institute convulsive precautions & do neurological status checks;
  • *pulmonary edema*: recognized by wet breath sounds, frothy, red-tinged mucus, increased BP, severe restlessness, cyanosis, distended neck veins, increased CVP; institute written emergency procedures for Rx of pulmonary edema, if one available in your unit; see NCPG #2:21, "Pulmonary Edema;"
  • *anemia*: due to decreased production of RBCs & an increased rate of hemolysis; manifested by dyspnea, pallor; blood transfusions should be given as frozen red cells to avoid antigenic stimulation of white cells & platelets (may also avoid transmission of hepatitis B &/or non-A, non-B hepatitis); regulate transfusion gtts/minute according to MD's orders.

4) Infection Control	The patient will remain free of hospital-based infections: — know that inflammatory responses & antibody production are decreased in ARF & wound healing is delayed; — no one with a cold or infection to enter pt.'s room; — turn pt. at least Q2H to prevent pulmonary complications; use blow bottles, coughing, & deep breathing PRN; — protect pt. from chilling & drafts; provide extra covers PRN; — take vital signs at least Q4H (sepsis may be present without febrile response); — keep any urinary drainage system a "closed system;" empty bag only PRN (once/shift); withdraw specimen with a sterile needle & syringe; indwelling catheter should be removed as soon as possible; — provide aseptic care of all wound & puncture sites; IV sites should be changed Q48–72H; — use "hepatitis precautions" (see NCPG #1:10, "The Patient with Hepatitis") to prevent cross contamination between pt. & staff; — provide scrupulous care of mouth at least Q4H & PRN; cleanse mouth with cotton applicators moistened with glycerin & lemon juice; use antiseptic mouthwashes; avoid stiff-bristled brushes because of tendency of gums to bleed.
5) Skin Integrity	The patient will be free of itchiness, skin redness, and uremic frost; patient's skin will be maintained as an excretory route for waste products: — know that daily dialysis as ordered by MD helps prevent itching, skin problems, & uremic frost; — bathe pt. at least daily & PRN to remove accumulated waste products; minimize use of soap; — if uremic frost develops, a weak vinegar solution (2 T of vinegar to 1 pt of warm water) may be used to dissolve deposited crystals; — apply lubricating lotions (without additives) to eliminate itchiness & dryness; — turn at least Q2H; use sheepskin protection for bony prominences & other standard decubitus-prevention measures.
6) Rest and Activity	The patient will be maintained in a rest and activity pattern that will provide comfort, decrease rate of metabolism, promote renal repair, and prevent loss of muscle mass: — pt. usually on complete bed rest; turn, position Q2H to avoid contractures & pressure; encourage ambulation as soon as possible; — have pt. take at least 5 deep breaths Q2H;

— provide for extended rest periods between activities such as eating, bathing, visitors, etc.;
— provide leg exercises or passive exercises Q4–8H to prevent loss of muscle mass & strength, & to prevent pulmonary embolus (see NCPGs #2:22, "Pulmonary Emboli," and #2:45, "Hazards of Immobility");
— try to maintain pt.'s normal day & night pattern of sleep.

7) Psychosocial Adjustment

The patient/family/SO will be provided with as much information about pt.'s condition as they need and want to know (in an effort to decrease usual anxieties and fears concomitant with an acute illness); the patient will be aided to return to independence:
— ask pt. what s/he is feeling & explain that patients usually have a variety of feelings, often the same as these (this will make pt. feel s/he is not unique or going crazy); allow pt. to express self freely; provide empathic listening;
— keep pt. informed of his progress, e.g., by interpreting lab results, vital signs, urinary output, etc.;
— explain purpose & sequence of all procedures & treatments & dialysis schedule; when pt. feels like it, have him participate as much as possible in own care;
— allow pt. to make as many decisions as possible regarding schedule, etc., in order to encourage independence;
— answer all questions as honestly as you can; pts. often have fears & questions about death & need to discuss it with someone; as a nurse, you are in a unique position to do this;
— give explanations & support to family &/or SO.

Discharge Planning and Teaching Objectives/Outcomes

1) (Patient/Family/Significant Other) Can verbalize cause, physiology, and treatment received for present illness.
2) Knows the role of all current medications, diet and discharge restrictions.
3) Knows the role of infection in kidney failure and preventive general health measures to carry out.
4) Has a schedule of permitted rest and activity periods, when and how to change them.
5) Knows early signs and symptoms of recurrence (see "Common Manifestations," page 1) and to report to doctor or clinic immediately.
6) Has an appointment to return to clinic or doctor's office for follow-up care.

Recommended References

"Bringing Them Back Out of Renal Shutdown," by J. Randolph. *RN*, May 1981:35–39, 108.

"BUN/Creatinine . . . Your Keys to Kidney Function," by J. Stark. *Nursing 80*, May 1980:33–38.

"Care of the Critically Ill Acute Renal Failure Patient," by J. Dory. *Critical Care Nurse*, November/December 1981:47–52.

"Catheters: Indwelling, Urinary." *NCP Guide #2:39*, 2nd Ed., Nurseco, 1980.

"Diet: Sodium-Restricted." *NCP Guide #3:44*, 2nd Ed., Nurseco, 1983.

"Drugs and Renal Disease," by M. Orr. *American Journal of Nursing*, May 1981:969–971.

"Fluids and Electrolytes, Parts A and B." *NCP Guides #3:48, 49*, 2nd Ed., Nurseco, 1983.

"Hazards of Immobility." *NCP Guide #2:45*, 2nd Ed., Nurseco, 1980.

"How to Succeed Against Acute Renal Failure," by J. Stark. *Nursing 82*, July 1982:26–33.

"Hyperalimentation." *NCP Guide #3:50*, 2nd Ed., Nurseco, 1983.

Nursing Management of Renal Problems, 2nd Ed., by D. Bundage. St. Louis: Mosby, 1980.

"The Patient on Dialysis." *NCP Guides #3:03–05*, 2nd Ed., Nurseco, 1983.

"The Patient with Hepatitis." *NCP Guide #1:10*, 2nd Ed., Nurseco, 1980.

"The Patient with Pulmonary Emboli." *NCP Guide #2:22*, 2nd Ed., Nurseco, 1980.

"Potassium Imbalance." *NCP Guide #1:10*, 2nd Ed., Nurseco, 1980.

'Renal Assessment: A Nursing Point of View," by S. Roberts. *Heart and Lung*, January/February 1979:105–113.

Standards of Clinical Practice: Acute Renal Failure. Pitman, NJ: American Association of Nephrology Nurses and Technicians (N. Woodbury Road, Box 56, 08071), 1982.

The Patient with Renal Failure: Chronic

Definition: Progressive deterioration of renal function that usually results in end stage renal disease necessitating dialysis or kidney transplant.

LONG TERM GOAL: The patient will maintain pre-dialysis status as long as possible, living within restrictions imposed by his disease, and will be able to deal with the possibility of long-term dialysis if necessary.

General Considerations:
— Read NCPG #3:13, "Acute Renal Failure."
— **Stages** of chronic renal failure (CRF):
   1) *diminished renal reserve*: reduced renal function without the accumulation of metabolic wastes in the blood;
   2) *renal insufficiency*: metabolic wastes begin to accumulate in blood; BUN, uric acid, serum creatinine, and phosphorus levels are elevated;
   3) *uremia*: excess amounts of nitrogenous wastes accumulate in the blood and the kidneys are unable to maintain homeostasis.
— **Onset** is usually slow with mild, intermittent symptoms such as headache, easy fatigability, anxiety, irritability, drowsiness, muscle twitching, uremic or toxic psychosis (hallucination, delusions), edema of peri-orbital, sacral, or peripheral areas, GI complaints. As condition progresses, symptoms increase in intensity due to accumulation of waste products in blood. Acidosis appears, as well as dehydration, increased anorexia and vomiting, muscle weakness, leg restlessness, and itching. CRF develops over months or years and is irreversible. Some type of maintenance dialysis is usually required; review NCPGs #3:03, "The Patient on Dialysis: Hemodialysis," and #3:05, "Dialysis: Peritoneal."
— **Treatment** aims include treating reversible causes of CRF (nephrotoxic agents, hypertension, sub-acute bacterial endocarditis, urinary tract infections, infectious diseases), implementing dietary and medical regimens for control of CRF, and treating associated cardiac conditions.
— **Nursing responsibilities** include providing patient and family teaching and counseling, keeping patient free of preventable complications, and preparing for access placement dialysis or kidney transplant when these options are exercised. This is accomplished by supplying patients with the necessary reading material to prepare them for the treatment modality. CRF patients have a high incidence of hepatitis B, non-A and non-B, due to multiple blood transfusions; staff awareness, precaution, and prevention should be practiced.

Specific Considerations, Potential Patient Outcomes, and Nursing Actions:

1) Fluids and Electrolytes

The patient will accept fluid restrictions in order to maintain fluid and electrolyte balance according to his individual needs; the patient will be free of preventable fluid and electrolyte imbalances:

— record I&O scrupulously & accurately; check with MD for amount of intake permitted; if possible, teach pt. to schedule own intake;

— weigh QD at same time, with same clothing & scale; use bed scale PRN; chart wt. (1 kg/2.2 lbs of wt. gain = 1 liter of retained fluid);

— pt. may be NPO; if so, provide mouth care at least Q4H & PRN;

— observe for signs & symptoms of fluid overload (engorged neck veins, increased body wt., tachycardia, increased BP & CVP, dyspnea, gallup rhythm, peripheral or cutaneous edema, rales); notify MD PRN;

— review NCPGs #3:48 & 49 ("Fluids & Electrolytes");

— know that blood levels of HCO_3 are often low, while NA, K & P levels may be high; know normal levels of serum electrolytes, check lab results & report to MD PRN.

2) Diet and Medications

The patient will adhere to dietary and medication regimens in order to decrease azotemia; the patient will maintain BUN, potassium, and phosphorus levels within acceptable limits:

— restrict protein intake as per MD's orders, usually 20–40 gms/day (normal protein intake is 55–60 gms/day);

— restrict Na, K, & fluid intake in an effort to prevent fluid accumulation, hypertension, & hyperkalemia; see NCPGs #2:48, "Potassium Imbalance" & #3:44, "Diet: Sodium-Restricted;"

— work with dietician to plan menus; if none available, refer to unit diet manuals, med-surg texts, or whatever sources are available;

— explain medical & dietary regimens to pt. so s/he may understand & adhere to them, even when experiencing side effects; share results & changes in blood chemistries, tests & correlate these with changes in diet & meds;

— involve pt. in menu selection & planning, include family; when able to follow dietary regimen in hospital, have pt. & family plan how they will follow it at home; have them make a written record of foods to include & exclude; teach them to read labels on canned goods for electrolyte content; locate low Na food items;

— teach pt. med schedule, purposes & effects of Q med; it is usually a priorty to keep serum Ca level at 9–10 mg/100 ml & phosphorous level below 6 mg/100 ml in order to prevent osteodystrophy; Vit. D is sometimes given to increase calcium absorption from the GI tract; antacids are frequently given;

— explain importance of antihypertensive meds & schedule, recognize & teach pt. S&S of hypotension & hypertension.

3) Infection Control

The patient will be maintained in an infection-free state; the patient will not contact secondary or hospital-based infections:
— know that these pts. have a low resistance to infections & that URIs are a particular hazard to them;
— wash hands *before* providing pt. care;
— turn, cough pt. (or use blow bottles) at least Q2H to prevent pulmonary complications; protect from drafts, chilling; provide extra covers PRN;
— take vital signs at least Q4H;
— carry out strict aseptic technique with burns, wounds, etc. to prevent sepsis;
— give strict aseptic catheter care; see NCPG #2:39, "Catheters: Indwelling Urethral;"
— review (with pt. & family) good general health measures to carry out at home.

4) Psychosocial Adjustment to Changes in Self-Image, Role Functioning

The patient will accept and adjust to body and role changes brought about by restrictions imposed by disease process; the patient will express, and staff will accept without judgment, any and all feelings, including negative ones and those dealing with death; the patient will be provided with information & rationale of treatment modalities:
— spend some time with pt. QD, discussing facts & concepts about his condition (preferably same nurse); ask him what this information means to him & how he feels about it; allow expression of any feelings, limiting only those that are destructive; refer to NCPGs #1:20–33, "Patient Behaviors;"
— know that adaptation may be a learned response & that pt. will go through the grief & mourning process; review NCPG #1:31, "Responses to Loss: the Grief & Mourning Process;"
— assess pt. motivation to adapt; ask pt. what his own goals are, work together to find ways s/he can meet them; because pt. is threatened with inability to carry out long-range life goals, focus on shorter-term ones;
— if a pt. feels hopeless & appears to refuse to adapt, s/he may express this by not adhering to prescribed regimes (may overindulge in food, fluids); review NCPGs #2:31 & #2:35, "Crisis Intervention;"
— discover pt.'s current ways of coping with stress; if they are working for him, support them; if not, help him find new alternatives by asking him what he thinks would make him feel better;
— discuss changes in usual role functioning & family relationships (often a problem if spouse has to go to work); include spouse & other family members in discussion; recommend family therapy or support groups PRN;

- if necessary, reorient pt. that his worth is not related to productivity; help him to focus on family relationships, e.g., nurturing his children, own independence;
- explain to pt. that usual & expected physical effects include feelings of lethargy & fatigue, drowsiness, generalized weakness, inability to function, weight loss, & changes in skin color (may be jaundiced or ashen blue);
- refer the pt. to appropriate source for assistance with financial problems;
- be aware that a pt. may refuse treatment to prolong own life; this is supported in the AHA's "Bill of Rights" for pts., which states a pt. has a right to do so after being informed of the consequences; continue emotional support to pt. & family if this decision is made;
- set up inservice conferences to discuss pt.'s rights, death & dying, adaptation to loss, & crisis intervention; this will help staff examine own feelings related to these subjects;
- refer the pt. to appropriate nephrology nurse specialist, transplant coordinator, or dialysis staff for detailed conferences about dialysis therapy &/or transplant;
- if you feel unable to help pt. with these psychosocial adjustments, find someone who can work with them (e.g., a psychiatric clinical specialist, psychiatrist, or other mental health worker); if none available in your facility, request one from the nearest community mental health center.

Discharge Planning and Teaching Objectives/Outcomes

1) (Patient/Family/Significant Other) Knows amount of daily fluid intake permitted and can plan schedule of intake; knows to weigh self daily, as a check on fluid retention, and to call doctor or clinic as indicated.
2) Has a written list of medications, dosages, schedules, and side effects, and knows to report appearance of latter.
3) Can select and plan own menu within dietary restrictions; has a written list of foods permitted and those to avoid.
4) Can explain relationship between infection and general preventive health measures; knows to call doctor or clinic at early signs of any infection, including URIs.
5) Can identify clinical manifestations that may indicate changes in fluid or electrolyte balance, and knows when to report these to doctor or clinic.
6) Can verbalize feelings about current condition, prognosis and treatment. Has access to continuing emotional support via individual, family, or group sessions, therapy, etc.
7) Has an appointment for access insertion (if appropriate).

Recommended References

"Access to the Bloodstream." *Review of Hemodialysis for Nurses and Dialysis Personnel.* St. Louis: Mosby, 1982:106–116.

"Adherence to the Prescribed Therapy for Chronic Renal Failure," by B. Ulrich. *Nephrology Nurse,* July/August 1981:14–21.

"Catheters: Indwelling Urethral." *NCP Guide #2:39,* 2nd Ed., Nurseco, 1980.

"Chronic Renal Failure." *Nursing Clinics of North America.* Philadelphia: Saunders, September 1981:487–597.

"Crisis Intervention." *NCP Guides #2:31, 35,* 2nd Ed., Nurseco, 1980.

"Dialysis Ambivalence: A Matter of Life & Death," by Diane & Daniel Auger. *American Journal of Nursing,* February 1976:276–277.

"Diet: Sodium-Restricted." *NCP Guide #3:44,* 2nd Ed., Nurseco, 1983.

"Fluids and Electrolytes: Parts A and B." *NCP Guides #3:48, 49,* 2nd Ed., Nurseco, 1983.

"Hemodialysis: Cannulas." *Development of Clinical Nephrology Practitioner,* by E. Larson, L. Lindbloom, and K. Davis. St. Louis: Mosby, 1982:200–206.

Living or Dying: Adaptation of Hemodialysis, by Norman B. Levy. Springfield, IL: Charles C. Thomas, 1974.

"Individualized Instruction for the Chronic Renal Failure Client," by S. Whitson. *Nephrology Nurse,* March/April 1982:12–18.

Nephrology Nursing (Perspectives of Care), by F. Hekelman and C. Ostendorp. New York: McGraw-Hill, 1979.

"Nutrition Notes," by B. Butler. *Nephrology Nurse,* September/October 1981:33–34.

"Patient Behaviors." *NCP Guides #1:20–33,* 2nd Ed., Nurseco, 1980.

Patient Care in Renal Failure, by J. Harrington & E. Brener. Philadelphia: Saunders, 1973.

"The Patient on Dialysis: Hemodialysis." *NCP Guide #3:03,* 2nd Ed., Nurseco, 1983.

"The Patient on Dialysis: Peritoneal." *NCP Guide #3:05,* 2nd Ed., Nurseco, 1983.

The Patient with End Stage Renal Disease, by L. Lancaster. New York: Wiley, 1979.

"The Patient Who is a Kidney Transplant Recipient." *NCP Guide #3:07,* 2nd Ed., Nurseco, 1983.

"The Patient in Renal Failure: Acute." *NCP Guide #3:13,* 2nd Ed., Nurseco, 1983.

"Potassium Imbalance." *NCP Guide #2:48,* 2nd Ed., Nurseco, 1980.

"Responses to Loss: The Grief and Mourning Process." *NCP Guide #1:31,* 2nd Ed., Nurseco, 1980.

"A Review of Hepatitis (Cause and Prevention) for Nephrology Nurses," by A. Corea. *Nephrology Nurse* May/June, 1979:17–22.

The Patient with a Total Hip Replacement

Definition: Total hip replacement (THR) surgery, also known as hip arthroplasty and hip prosthesis, involves removal of diseased hip bone tissue followed by replacement of the acetabulum with a plastic cup and the head of the femur with a steel ball and stem. Prosthetic devices vary considerably and the selection is the choice of the surgeon based on research findings, his own experience, and the special needs of a particular patient.

LONG TERM GOAL: The patient will recover from successful reconstructive hip surgery free of preventable complications, returning to home/family/community roles and responsibilities while adapting to a regimen of exercise and increased activity appropriate to stage of convalescence and general health status.

General Considerations:

— **Indications** for surgery include degenerative hip joint changes caused by arthritis and congenital anomalies, increasing difficulty walking, and increasing pain experiences.

— **Surgery** aims to remove diseased bone tissue, to replace needed parts, and to improve mobility and activity potential with the relief of pain. Patients with either unilateral or bilateral THR can expect a significant increase in walking cadence, stride length, and speed without the need for assistive aids. The greatest improvement will be seen in the three months to one year recovery period, although total gains will still be below a normal walking efficiency and gait pattern. By hospital discharge, in less than three weeks, the patient is afebrile and ambulatory, bearing weight with elbow crutches, walker, or cane temporarily; the wound is usually healed and patient needs only mild oral medication for discomfort. Depending on the type of work and the patient's condition, some can return to work in eight to twelve weeks. Many patients are middle-aged, but most are over 65 years of age. Refer, if necessary, to NCPG #2:33, "The Aged Patient: Physiology of Aging."

— **Preoperatively,** the patient receives a complete history and physical exam, including EKG, x-rays (AP and lateral of chest, pelvis, affected leg, abductions of leg and hip), and laboratory studies (CBC, SGOT, sed rate, serum electrolytes, type and cross-match). Pre- and postoperative venous flow studies to locate occlusions may also be done. The surgeon also takes time to explain thoroughly the expected operative procedure and anticipated rehabilitation plan.

— **Nursing responsibilities** include pre-op patient preparation (assessment, care, and teaching), post-op care (prevention of complications, positioning, and exercise), and patient discharge planning and teaching.

Specific Considerations, Potential Patient Outcomes, and Nursing Actions:

1) Pre-op
   Preparation
The patient indicates s/he understands the nature of hip condition, proposed surgery, and rehabilitation regimen; the patient expresses an optimistic, realistic, and reasonable expectation of a successful surgical outcome; the patient will be physiologically and psychologically stabilized and prepared for surgery:
   — using audiovisual methods, explain the orthopedic procedure, devices, & rehabilitation regimen to pt. & family;
   — know that these pts. are often fearful even though they want the operation; provide them with needed encouragement, reassurance, & repeated simple explanations;
   — explain the importance of & show pt. post-op positioning (toes pointed upward, legs abducted), turning & traction set-up (if one will be used), & the type of abduction splint that will be used;
   — teach gluteal & quadriceps muscle-setting exercises along with knee & ankle flexion exercises; teach coughing & deep breathing exercises; have pt. return demonstrations correctly;
   — obtain informed written consents for surgery & anesthesia;
   — assist in the provision of a useful data base for post-op evaluation of pt.'s status;
   — refer to NCPG #2:44, "General Pre-Op Care," for additional appropriate nursing actions;
   — prep pt. from nipples to mid-calf; have pt. take shower with antibacterial soap; have pt. scrub gently skin of operative hip for 20 minutes using Phisohex, Betadine, or similar preparation (this may be done 3 times pre-op: 24 hours prior to surgery, 12 hours pre-op, and the morning of surgery);
   — apply Ace bandages or TED Hose (if ordered) from toe to knee or toe to hip, according to surgeon preference;
   — administer prophylactic antibiotics & preanesthetic medications as ordered;
   — perform other standard preoperative preparations indicated for this pt.

2) Post-op
   Positioning
The patient will maintain the prescribed post-op position for functional healing of the hip joint without dislocation; the patient will be free of circulatory status complications:
   — prepare pt.'s bed with firm mattress, bed board, overhead trapeze, & frame with traction for the affected leg, adjustable footboard for the unaffected leg, bed rails, & a sheepskin; take bed to recovery room or OR; refer to NCPG #2:50, "Traction: General Principles;"
   — know that pt. position, type of leg traction, & turning may vary according to surgical approach (*although hip abduction is always maintained* & excessive hip flexion is avoided); sometimes a pillow or foam wedge is strapped

between legs with Velcro straps to maintain abduction; make certain *all* care providers understand the prescribed leg position & method of patient movement; maintain proper alignment & position at *all times*;
— observe for & report sharp hip pain promptly, as hip may have dislocated & a return to OR may be necessary.

3) Prevention of Complications

The patient will be free of preventable complications (or have them promptly managed and controlled); the patient will maintain effective normal body functions:
— refer to applicable nursing actions in NCPGs #2:41–43, "General Post-Op Care, Part A: Support of Pulmonary Functions; Part B: Support of Cardiovascular Functions; Part C: Support of Auxiliary Functions;"
— observe for signs & symptoms of complications specific to this surgery:
  a) *excessive bleeding*
  • monitor vital signs Q15 minutes as ordered & determined advisable;
  • measure & record Hemovac contents at least Q8H until removed;
  • observe dressing; report excessive bleeding; apply pressure dressing PRN;
  b) *pressure sores*
  • give skin care to back & pressure points Q2H;
  • use appropriate decubitus-prevention measures/devices; refer to NCPG #4:42, "Decubitus Ulcer Care: Prevention & Treatment;"
  c) *wound infection*
  • reinforce or change dry sterile dressing using strict aseptic technique;
  • observe & record skin color, temperature, integrity, appearance at least Q8H;
  • observe & report wound redness, warmth, odor, or drainage; note rising sed rate or WBC;
  • notify MD of temp elevations above 38°C (100.4°F) 5 days or more post-op;
  • administer antibiotics prophylactically as ordered;
  d) *peroneal nerve palsy*
  • monitor & record nerve function & circulation on affected leg Q1H 1st 24 hours; Q2H 2nd 24 hours & as advisable after that; refer to NCPG #2:50, "Traction: General Principles," for assessment parameters;
  e) *thrombo-embolus*
  • avoid pillows & pads *under* knees or calves;
  • have pt. flex toes, feet, & ankles Q1H.

| 4) Rest and Exercise | The patient will strengthen hip muscles and begin progressive weight-bearing ambulation; the patient will remain free of flexion contractures, dislocation of hip prosthesis, or thrombo-embolitic episodes: |

- ask pt. to contract & relax gluteal & quadriceps muscles about 10x/H when awake; observe & record that this is being done; teach pt. that these exercises improve venous blood return to heart as well as maintain & strengthen leg muscle tone in readiness for walking;
- assist pt. in transfers to walker & chair, bearing weight gradually on affected leg *as permitted*; get pt. out of bed on operative side, elevate head of bed 45°, & have pt. grasp trapeze, while you support legs with abductor foam splint securely in place;
- while pt. is sitting, maintain hip abduction with pillows; avoid hip flexion by propping pt. in a semi-reclining position (70°);
- transport pt. in prone position via stretcher to PT twice daily when ordered; observe & support PT exercise & gait training program;
- when allowed BRP, have pt. use a raised toilet seat; until then, have pt. push with good leg & lift with trapeze to get on an orthopedic bed pan.

Discharge Planning and Teaching Objectives/Outcomes

1) (Patient/Family/Significant Other) Can state restrictions for affected leg, i.e., need to use a cane, walker, or crutches temporarily for support and partial weight-bearing ambulation; the type of chair to be used and the kind of sitting posture to assume as well as the length of total daily sitting time; the need to avoid hip hyperflexion, bending, twisting, stooping, crossing legs, and lifting heavy objects; the need to rotate hips laterally when putting on socks and shoes; the need to avoid sleeping on the *operative* side for up to two months post-op; understands that a newly replaced hip joint can dislocate during first three months, so care must be taken to follow instructions faithfully.

2) States s/he knows to report promptly to doctor any signs of wound drainage, pain in leg or chest, calf tenderness, or coughing up blood; indicates s/he will wear elastic stockings during daytime hours for as long as doctor wishes.

3) Knows and expresses willingness to follow home exercise program and general health measures, adjusting to normal activities gradually as condition permits; after a three-month rehabilitation period, will consider taking up recreational exercise in the form of walking, cycling, or swimming because s/he knows that weight on the hip joint is lessened in the latter two activities and that the risk of prosthesis loosening is very small.

4) Has name and phone number of community resources to be contacted PRN (social security disability, home health service, senior citizens services, or other).

5) Has written set of instructions for all of the above.

Recommended References

"The Aged Patient: Physiology of Aging." *NCP Guide #2:33*, 2nd Ed., Nurseco, 1980.

"Decubitus Ulcer Care: Prevention and Treatment." *NCP Guide #4:42*, 2nd Ed., Nurseco, 1983.

"General Post-op Care, Parts A, B, and C." *NCP Guides #2:41–43*, 2nd Ed., Nurseco, 1980.

"General Pre-op Care." *NCP Guide #2:44*, 2nd Ed., Nurseco, 1980.

"Preoperative Education for the Total Hip Patient," by M. Mattix. *Orthopedic Nurses Association Journal*, June 1979:251–252.

"Traction: General Principles." *NCP Guide #2:50*, 2nd Ed., Nurseco, 1980.

The Child with Asthma

Definition: Asthma is an intermittent and reversible obstructive condition of the small bronchioles resulting from constriction of bronchial smooth muscle, mucosal edema, excessive production of mucus, and the interplay of various immunological mechanisms.

LONG TERM GOAL: The child will achieve optimal health through a balanced program of rest and exercise, proper nutrition, management of physical and emotional stress, avoidance of precipitants to an asthmatic attack, and appropriate medication regimen, if indicated.

General Considerations:

— **Incidence:** 8 million Americans, of which over 1.5 million are school age children.

— The **underlying mechanism** for most asthmatic children is an *allergic response* to a specific antigen. Food allergies are common in infants; inhalants are the usual offenders in older children. Precipitants range from pollens, dust, odors, fumes, smoke, animal hair, molds, foods, and yellow food coloring to infections, emotional stress, cold air, hot and dry winds, seasonal changes, and/or vigorous activity.

— **Contact with a precipitant** causes the bronchioles to go into spasm and constriction, the mucous membranes to become edematous and produce thick mucus, and the obstructed airway to trap air in the alveoli, thereby altering the free exchange of blood gases.

— **Onset of an attack** may follow an emotionally or physically traumatic experience or may occur at night while the child is sleeping. Attacks may last from a few hours to a few days, leaving the child exhausted. *Gradual onset* of an asthmatic attack may be indicated with sneezing, nasal congestion, and a slight cough; *sudden onset* of an acute attack is characterized by rapid and shallow breathing, paroxysmal coughing, expiratory wheezing, rales, thick and tenacious mucus, elevated heart rate, anxiety and fear bordering on panic, and restlessness. Without prompt measures to dilate bronchioles and alleviate symptoms, the process progresses to severe hypoxemia (associated with complaints of headache, fatigue, confusion, dizziness) and increased carbon dioxide retention (associated with drowsiness, diaphoresis, muscular twitching, waning consciousness). Medical emergency measures must immediately be used to combat impending respiratory failure.

— **Diagnosis** is based on a thorough history and physical, chest x-ray, eosinophil count of sputum, nasal secretions, and peripheral blood samples, skin testing, arterial blood gas determinations, and spirometric pulmonary function tests. A bronchial challenge test measures the response inside the respiratory system to substances inhaled under controlled conditions. Peak expiratory flow rate (PEFR) meter readings and data recordings provide information to help determine bronchodilator drug usage according to severity of condition and need.

— **Treatment** is symptomatic during acute episodes, consisting of humidified oxygen, increased oral and IV hydration, appropriate drugs (bronchodilators, expectorants, and, if necessary, antibiotics or corticosteroids), and stress-reducing environmental management. Long-term therapy to prevent recurrences includes: removing the offending allergen(s), desensitization measures, normalization of respiratory function (via drugs, physical therapy, selected sports), and development of a personalized, effective, therapeutic regimen that both child and parent understand and accept.

— **Status asthmaticus** is a condition of a severe asthmatic's failure to respond to appropriate drug therapy. Prompt medical management includes: balancing fluid & electrolyte status; monitoring CVP and vital signs; administering humidified oxygen, IPPB, and chest physiotherapy; and augmenting drug therapy to include antibiotics for infection and corticosteroids.

— **Nursing responsibilities** involve, primarily, assistance to the parents and child in the prevention and control of asthma, both during and after hospitalization. Review NCPGs #3:22–26, "Normal Growth & Development," for appropriate age level; refer to Recommended References for additional information.

Specific Considerations, Potential Patient Outcomes, and Nursing Actions:

1) Respiratory Distress

The child will resume a normal breathing pattern, will maintain a patent airway, and will expectorate loosened secretions:

— observe, record, & report pattern, rate, & characteristics of respiration;
— chart frequency, amount, & appearance of expectorated sputum; save specimen for lab analysis;
— assess cardiac status, skin, & nailbed color, vital signs;
— place child in a sitting position of comfort to provide greater chest expansion; support with pillows or padded overbed table to lean on;
— administer humidified O_2 at prescribed flow rate to maintain arterial pO_2 at 65–100 (cyanosis appears in children with a pO_2 less than 55–65); use of mist tents are controversial as they are believed to provoke bronchoconstriction, so, unless otherwise ordered, administer O_2 via nasal catheter; avoid face masks because of smothering sensation they cause & because they interfere with expectorating sputum;
— increase oral intake to help loosen & liquify sputum; give warm or room temperature liquids because cold fluids may cause coughing spasms;

— administer IV fluids (usually 1500 to 3000 ml/m² of body surface Q24H), watch for IV infiltration; monitor I&O; record urine specific gravity findings, & observe for signs of fluid overload; weigh daily; review lab reports;
— avoid sedatives, tranquilizers, analgesics such as morphine & antihistamines that depress the respiration & cough reflex;
— assist PT & RPT in postural drainage & inhalation therapy; learn techniques of positioning, coughing, percussion, vibration, & segmental breathing to reinforce teaching of child & parents;
— observe for early signs of respiratory failure during acute attacks (decreasing pO_2, increasing pCO_2, changes in inspiratory breath sounds, increased use of accessory muscles of respiration, increasingly high pitched expiratory wheezing (although with very little airflow & worsening condition wheezing may be minimal or not present), & waning consciousness);
— report deteriorating condition STAT; have readily available endotracheal tubes, laryngoscope, tracheostomy equipment, volume-cycled ventilator, & drug stimulants for immediate emergency use;
— during periods of respiratory comfort, offer foods in small amts that are soft, high caloric, easily digestible, & age appropriate.

2) Medications   The child will experience symptomatic relief via medications; the child will help the nurse assess own response to medications:
— know & teach the action, dosage range, storage, administration, side effects, & contraindications for all drugs administered; refer to NCPG #2:36, "Drugs: Asthma," as well as accompanying literature supplied with medication;
— stay with child while meds are taken; be direct & honest in answering questions about meds; mask unpleasant-tasting drugs with honey, syrup, or desired drink; obtain adequate assistance for child's protection while administering parenteral meds;
— observe, record, & report child's response to medication; elicit cooperation & contributions from parents & child; pay particular attention to evaluation for possible drug interactions when giving more than one kind of medication;
— teach child & parents that caffeine products (cola drinks, chocolate, coffee, tea) should be avoided as they tend to aggravate the nervousness caused by ephedrine or theophylline preparations;
— to facilitate precise dosage administration, teach parents & children to use dram-marked containers, rather than teaspoons, & to store all medications in tightly closed containers away from light & heat.

3) Anxiety and Fear

The child will stay calm and respond appropriately to fearful situations; the child will integrate asthmatic experiences into a positive self-concept:
- provide an accessible call bell for child; establish a trusting relationship that is frequently reinforced by visits to check on child, by talking, by touching, by manner & attitude while giving care to child;
- teach child to use diaphragm, rather than just lungs, to pull in & expel deep breaths of air when s/he first feels a tightening sensation in chest; demonstrate to child & parent how deep breathing, slowly, can induce relaxation & calm;
- teach child & parent how to control their panic with first signs of asthmatic attack, e.g., to visually imagine staying calm & under control, to begin slow, deep breathing exercises, to sip warm water;
- *never* leave child alone during an acute attack; if parental anxiety is too high, it would be better for pt. if someone who is calm & supportive be with him; work with parent until parent can be a calming influence;
- hold child in an upright position & rock him (as effective as bedrest if a relaxed, confident approach is used);
- reduce the level of non-productive stimuli by keeping room quiet, dimming lighting; use soft music to induce relaxation & rest;
- when an acute attack is over, assess factors that precipitated attack; answer the pt.'s questions about his condition factually & encourage a positive familial interaction by including parents in pt.'s care & discharge planning;
- allow pt. to meet own needs as condition improves by keeping frequently used items in easy reach, by being available, but not overprotective, & by encouraging resumption of normal patterns of living;
- provide child with tasks at which s/he can be successful; praise all efforts; explain to parents the importance of successful experiences in promoting positive self-image;
- consider occupational therapy for the older child & utilize play therapy for younger child to provide age-appropriate diversion during hospitalization; refer to NCPG #3:30, "Play Therapy: General Suggestions."

4) Prevention of Recurrences, Child/ Family Education

The child will be free of secondary infections; the child will integrate a balanced program of rest, exercise, nutrition, prescribed medications, and physical therapy into daily routine; the child and parents will try to avoid offending allergens and attack-precipitating factors in regular environment:
- implement allergen-free hospital environment & discuss with child & family what modifications can be made at home;
- organize nursing care to provide adequate rest periods; discuss with parents need for periodic rest periods to avoid excessive fatigue & lowered resistance;

— identify possible precipitating factors with child & family; teach child & parent how to avoid or cope with stressful experiences;

— stress importance of hydration at all times: during play, before & after exercise, in warm weather or overheated room in winter, when teething or afflicted with colds, sore throats, fevers, or other illnesses;

— urge parents to see MD regularly & at the first indication of a respiratory infection or asthmatic attack;

— assess family members' feelings & reactions to asthmatic child (e.g., overprotection, overanxiety, frustration, resentment, anger, guilt, depression, helplessness); provide opportunities for recognition & acceptance of these negative feelings; listen to parents discuss problems & support them in working out their own best solutions; refer family for counseling PRN;

— know that failure of treatment is directly related to level of compliance with prescribed medical regimen & that compliance is associated with a high level of understanding & acceptance of the nature of the asthmatic condition, how the medication works, how precipitants need to be controlled, & how important chest physical therapy is to prevent & control attacks;

— teach child to begin slow, deep breathing exercises & to sip warm water when symptoms of an attack are beginning to occur;

— encourage lung-developing types of exercises & games (e.g., jogging, soccer, swimming); for children with musical ability, playing a wind instrument can develop lungs & produce relaxation from tension; encourage summer camp experience;

— provide literature on asthma & review with parent.

Discharge Planning and Teaching Objectives/Outcomes

1) (Parent/Guardian (and child when able)) States s/he knows the importance of good nutrition and allowing sufficient time for eating smaller meals, several times daily.
2) Can identify situation or agents that precipitate an asthmatic attack and will conscientiously try to avoid these.
3) Recognizes signs of an impending attack (cough, wheezing, fever, N&V, increased anxiety or tension) and knows the steps to take to minimize distress (position, rest, medications, fluids, visualization).
4) States s/he understands the importance of both rest and exercise, and can help plan activities around a sensible schedule.
5) Can state the individual medications and treatments required, possible side effects, purposes, amount, and indications for administration.
6) States s/he knows to prevent exposure to infections and to seek prompt medical care for these and for unrelieved attacks.

7) Knows resources for obtaining more information about asthma:
   American Lung Association (branches in major cities), 1740 Broadway, New York, NY 10019
   Asthma & Allergy Foundation of America, 19 W. 44th St., New York, NY 10036
   National Foundation for Asthma, Inc., P.O. Box 50304, Tucson, AZ 85703
   National Jewish Hospital/National Asthma Center, Dept. of Pediatrics, 3800 E. Colfax Ave., Denver, CO 80206
8) Has a referral to a home health agency for assistance in assessing and modifying the home environment as needed to control allergens.

Recommended References

"A Prescription for Compliance . . . an Asthmatic Child and His Parents." *Emergency Medicine*, February 29, 1980:73–74.

"Acute and Chronic Asthma: A Guide to Intervention," by D. Hudgel and L. Madsen. *American Journal of Nursing*, October 1980:1791–1795.

"Assessment of the Individual with Altered Respiratory Function," by J. Rokosky. *Nursing Clinics of North America*, June 1981:195–207.

Asthma. Denver: National Asthma Center (3800 E. Colfax, 80206).

Better Living and Breathing (A Manual for Patients), 2nd Ed., by K. Moser et al. St. Louis: Mosby, 1980.

"Breathing Exercises as Play for Asthmatic Children," by H. McCaully. *MCN: American Journal of Maternal Child Nursing*, September/October 1980:340–344.

Breathing Exercises for Asthmatic Children. Evanston, IL: American Academy of Pediatrics (PO Box 1034, 60204).

"Drugs: Asthma." *NCP Guide #2:36*, 2nd Ed., Nurseco, 1980.

"Normal Growth & Development: Newborn to Adolescent." *NCP Guides #3:22–26*, 2nd Ed., Nurseco, 1983.

"Play Therapy: General Suggestions." *NCP Guide #3:30*, 2nd Ed., Nurseco, 1983.

Super Stuff (Kit for elementary school age child). New York: The American Lung Association (19 W. 44th St., 10019).

Teaching Myself About Asthma, by Parcel et al. St. Louis: Mosby, 1979.

"The Asthmatic Child: Preventing and Controlling Attacks," by R. Wieczorek and B. Horner-Rosner. *American Journal of Nursing*, February 1979:258–262.

The Child with Diarrhea

Definition: Diarrhea is an increase in the volume, fluidity, or frequency of bowel movements relative to the usual habit of each individual. Diarrhea is a symptom of a pathophysiological process within the intestinal tract, not a disease itself.

LONG TERM GOAL: The child will regain normal intestinal motility and function essential to continued growth and well-being; the patient will return to a level of health associated with the re-establishment of fluid and electrolyte balance followed by a return to normal dietary intake.

General Considerations:
— Diarrhea is considered "acute" if it is less than one week in duration; "subacute" type lasts one to two weeks, and "chronic" diarrhea refers to cases lasting longer than two weeks.
— **Causes:** most commonly viral gastroenteritis; also bacterial and parasitic infections, drugs, dietary allergies, excitement, or stress.
— Infants and toddlers are the most vulnerable to diarrheal infections. They have the poorest compensatory mechanisms to counteract dehydration, electrolyte disturbances, and pathogenic invaders.
— **Physiological disturbances** related to diarrhea center around dehydration, metabolic acidosis, and shock. Clinical manifestations in *mild* cases include: a low grade fever, vomiting, gastrointestinal irritability, and two to ten loose stools per day; *severe diarrhea* manifests the above signs plus anorexia, a weight loss of 10% or more, abdominal distention and cramping, poor skin turgor with dry mucous membranes, a rapid and weak pulse, deep respirations, and a diminishing output; if onset is sudden, the patient may have a temperature of 40–41° C (104–106°F).
— **Treatment** aims to eliminate the causative agent (when known), reduce oral intake of solid foods, replace fluids and electrolytes, and re-establish a normal gastrointestinal intake and output. For dietary management, see NCPG #3:43, "Diet: Diarrhea Control."
— **Nursing responsibilities** include assessment of the child's hydration status, physical condition, and pertinent history; implementation of fluid replacement and dietary measures; evaluation of the child's response to treatment; and parent/guardian education regarding resumption of care at home and prevention of further diarrheal episodes.
— Review NCPGs #3:22–26, "Normal Growth and Development," for appropriate age level.

Specific Considerations, Potential Patient Outcomes, and Nursing Actions:
1) Fluids and Electrolytes   The patient will regain a normal fluid and electrolyte balance and meet nutritional requirements:
— refer to NCPGs #3:48 & 49, "Fluid & Electrolyte Balance;"

— know signs of increasing dehydration (changes in skin turgor, depressed fontanels, sunken eyes, weight loss, rapid pulse, decreasing urine output); observe for them & report to MD;

— monitor IV hourly; regulate fluids through an IVAC or volume control method according to MD's orders; restrain pt. PRN to maintain patency of IV; check for infiltration; refer to NCPG #2:24, "Intravenous Therapy;"

— reduce insensible fluid loss (via skin & lungs) by decreasing temp elevations with tepid sponge baths, meds as ordered, & minimal clothing;

— weigh pt. daily or more frequently if necessary to monitor fluid losses; record I&O accurately;

— follow lab reports daily & compare them with pt.'s clinical appearance to verify response;

— keep pt. NPO to rest bowel (usually ordered for 12–48 hours); resume oral intake gradually, using sterile water or an electrolyte solution & progressing from half-strength to full strength; depending on the causative agent, a previous diet may need to be changed; toleration of new diets or reappearance of diarrhea must be promptly & accurately reported; refer to NCPG #3:43, "Diet: Diarrhea Control."

2) Infection Control

The patient will be free of secondary infection; the infectious organism will be identified and controlled, when possible:

— use strict handwashing techniques when handling pt., diapers, or bedding; know that full isolation precautions are usually not necessary; use disposable diapers & bed protectors;

— report cases of shigella & salmonella to local health dept. for epidemiologic follow-up;

— during acute phase, test all stools for blood, sugar, protein; send specimen to lab for culture, ova, & parasites;

— record vital signs Q4H & report abnormalities;

— record & report changes in stool frequency, consistency, or pattern; report increasing signs of dehydration or shock; record urine specific gravity Q4H;

— give meds sparingly & only as ordered, since they can mask the intensity of the disease, especially in young children; know that they may also retard the elimination of toxins or other pathogenic materials; know that absorbents such as kaolin or pectin may provide consistency to a watery stool, but should not be used over a week as they may absorb nutrients;

— know that yogurt & other lactobacilli preparations may be ordered to help re-establish normal intestinal flora with prolonged diarrhea symptoms following antibiotic treatment;

— instruct parent/guardian in the proper method of making, storing, & giving formula & meals; reinforce with demonstrations of effective handwashing technique & sanitation habits; have parents do correct return demonstrations.

3) Comfort   The child will be comfortable and will fulfill maturational needs for trust, warmth, security:
- take time for physical & verbal contact at least hourly; stroke & comfort, especially when parents or others are unavailable to stay with child;
- meet the need for oral sucking satisfaction in the young infant & child with a pacifier or teething toy; burp child PRN to expel swallowed air;
- reposition pt. Q2–3H, remove IV restraints, & place extremities through range of motion exercises to promote circulation & to allow pt. periods of supervised freedom;
- moisten lips & mouth with glycerin swabs or a cool damp cloth frequently, to prevent cracked lips & dryness;
- relieve some abdominal cramping by placing a warm cloth on the abdomen, changing position, & holding pt. to minimize crying (will reduce the amount of swallowed air that adds to distention).

Discharge Planning and Teaching Objectives/Outcomes:

1) (Patient/Guardian) Can state how to prevent a recurrence, identifying relevant causes and remedy.
2) Say they understand the importance of keeping child well hydrated.
3) Will keep child isolated from possible sources of infection.
4) Recognize danger signs of diarrhea (more than three to four loose stools, loss of appetite, fever, vomiting, change in breathing, diminished urination) and the need for prompt medical care.
5) Will notify pediatric clinic or public health nurse if symptoms are not gone in one week or if there are repeated episodes of diarrhea over a period of weeks or months.

Recommended References

"Acute Diarrheal Infections in Infants' Prospects for Immunoprophylaxis. Part I Bacterial and Viral Causes," by M. Levine and R. Edelman. *Hospital Practice*, December 1979:89-91, 94-100. Part II, *Hospital Practice*, January 1980:97-104.

"Diet: Diarrhea Control." *NCP Guide #3:43*, 2nd Ed., Nurseco, 1983.

"Feeding Infants with Diarrhea." *Emergency Medicine*, March 30, 1981:111.

"Fluid & Electrolytes." *NCP Guides #3:48, 49*, 2nd Ed., Nurseco, 1983.

"Home Care for Diarrhea" (Patient Education Aid). *Patient Care*, March 15, 1981:163.

"Intravenous Therapy: General Principles." *NCP Guide #2:46*, 2nd Ed., Nurseco, 1980.

"Normal Growth & Development: Newborn to Adolescent." *NCP Guides #3:22-26*, 2nd Ed., Nurseco, 1983.

"Sodium and Water Content of Feedings for Use in Infants with Diarrhea," by S. Walker et al. *Clinical Pediatrics*, March 1981:199-204.

"The Relationship of Oral Rehydration Solution to Hypernatremia in Infantile Diarrhea," by T.G. Cleary et al. *Journal of Pediatrics*, November 1981:739-741.

The Child with Epilepsy

Definition: Epilepsy is a convulsive-type disorder of the nervous system characterized by sudden and periodic lapses of consciousness known as seizures.

LONG TERM GOAL: The child will lead a relatively normal life, participating in social and athletic activities; the child will be seizure-free due to medication, but will understand and accept the reality of his possibly life-long condition; the child will cope effectively with feelings of self-worth and self-confidence consistent with realistic educational and career goals.

General Considerations:
— **Incidence and occurrence:** 73 of 100,000 children under age one; similar incidence up to age 10, then dropping off; most children outgrow condition by adulthood and nearly three out of four are seizure-free after stopping medication. Disorder occurs in both sexes, any race.
— **Seizure Classification—International:** refer to NCPG #3:06, "The Patient with Epilepsy."
— Petit mal, or absence, seizures are more common in children six to fourteen years old and often disappear after puberty. Seizures can occur 100 times a day and often go unnoticed.
— **Causes:** the electrical disturbance of the brain may be caused by a single factor, a combination of factors, or be unknown. Causes are numerous and include metabolic disturbances, cerebral trauma, brain lesions, CNS infections, and ingestion of toxic drugs or chemicals. Not all seizures indicate epilepsy; some are related to fever, electrolyte imbalance, hypoglycemia, or an acute infection. Seizures may be precipitated, in those with a lower seizure threshold, by fatigue, stress, malnutrition, or trauma.
— **Low birth weight babies** have considerable seizure activity, especially those who had hypoxic episodes before or during delivery. These may resolve only to show up as athetoid cerebral palsy or other cerebral palsy involvement. In another form of seizure activity, infants may develop a myoclonic type of seizure at three to four months with gradual deterioration of development. Treatment sometimes lessens seizures but often without improvement in growth and development rate. These children are generally not called "epileptic," since epilepsy usually is considered an episodic event or disorder in an otherwise healthy individual. For pediatric nurses however, contact with seizuring infants is more apt to fit these categories. See Recommended References for additional information.
— **Adolescents with epilepsy** are especially vulnerable to seizures in conditions of menstruation, alcohol or drug abuse, pregnancy, and large weight gains or losses.

— **Diagnosis** is based on a thorough history, complete physical and neurological examination with a battery of tests including skull x-rays, brain scan, angiography, pneumoencephalogram, and electroencephalogram (EEG). See Recommended References to prepare patient for an EEG.

— **Treatment** aims to control or minimize seizures via medication; to remove or control any known causes of seizure activity; to establish good general health with normal growth and development; and to promote a balanced, moderate, fairly normal, and active childhood with self-acceptance and self-esteem.

— **Nursing responsibilities** include assisting with diagnosis and treatment plan; providing seizure precautions and prevention of injury; teaching and counseling child/family re: reality of epilepsy, acceptance and compliance with continuing medical regimen, and preparation to assume self-confident self or child care; assisting the child and family to cope with social stigma and rejection; and consulting with child's school teacher, nurse, and principal re: child's condition and care, first aid for seizures, classmate acceptance and help, misconceptions and prejudices about seizure disorders. The nurse should provide parents and school with appropriate literature from local or national epilepsy organization; see Recommended References for suggestions. Epilepsy clinical nurse specialists are now available in some medical centers and may be consulted for nursing staff development and community education programs.

— **Status epilepticus** (SE) is a condition of prolonged seizures or rapid, successive seizures; it is a medical emergency because death can result from anoxia or exhaustion. Some 5–10% of the pediatric population has SE at some time; half of these are under the age of two. Mortality rate can be as high as 50%; death results primarily from cardiac and respiratory arrest. Immediate treatment will be concerned with maintaining an airway and vital functions, protecting child from harm, drawing blood for lab tests, starting an IV infusion, and giving glucose with antiepileptic drugs. Valproic acid (VAL or Depakene) is now being used successfully for treating refractory seizures. VAL tends to decrease serum phenytoin (Dilantin) and elevate serum phenobarbital, but not with predictable certainty. Combination drug therapy must therefore include continuing and close monitoring of all serum drug concentrations.

Specific Considerations, Potential Patient Outcomes, and Nursing Actions:

1) Seizure Precautions — The patient will sustain no injuries and will not aspirate tongue, mucus, or foreign objects; the child's seizure will be controlled as safely and as soon as possible; the child's seizures will be accurately observed, described, and documented; the child will regain postictal reorientation and stable condition:

— remain calm, reassuring, matter-of-fact, since attitudes influence behavior of onlookers, both children & adults;

— keep bed rails up & padded when child is in bed; explain to child & obtain cooperation;

— check vital signs & level of consciousness Q2H; observe & report unusual behavior;

— tape plastic oral airway (for possible use by physician or qualified nurse) in one clearly designated, easily accessible place (usually head of bed) & have an alternate on the pt. when s/he leaves room for diagnostic tests or other reasons; know that *first aid* measures for lay people specifically indicate that tongue blades or other objects should NOT be placed in a seizuring child's mouth;

— label all x-ray, lab, & off-nursing-unit situation requests with "SEIZURE PRECAUTIONS" in red ink;

— hold conferences for nursing staff, auxiliary medical personnel, parents, as well as child's friends re: this pt.'s particular type of seizure (once it has been fully described & identified) & the safe, appropriate first aid care measures to be provided during & after a seizure; tell parents of the need to provide this information to child's teacher & school administration office (since school nurse is usually not available); provide parent with First Aid for Seizure leaflets and School Alert Kit to take to school officials (see Recommended References);

— take only rectal or axillary temperatures & notify all nursing staff of this precautionary measure;

— have readily accessible for immediate use: oxygen & suction equipment, IV supplies, parenteral antiepileptic drugs (more than one type: diazepam, phenobarbital, phenytoin, VAL), cardiac & respiratory stimulants, & IV bicarbonate;

— never leave child alone once a seizure begins; if possible, place child in a supine, side-lying position; loosen clothing at neck & waist; remove glasses; protect head with your arms, lap, cushion, or safe substitute; protect child from environmental dangers (furniture, walls, equipment, etc.);

— for complex partial seizures, do not try to stop purposeless behavior & do not touch, annoy, or argue with a child out of control; urge onlookers to leave scene, assuring them that you will cope with situation;

— maintain an open airway by extending neck, turning face to side if possible; intubate with oral airway if available & in your judgment indicated; do not force anything between clenched teeth; suction secretions PRN;

— remain with child until fully conscious & reoriented or until you have determined child to be in stable condition although asleep; allow child to rest or sleep after seizure; know that child may also display incoherent speech, extreme restlessness, &/or confusion for which s/he is not responsible after a seizure & that this condition may persist for minutes or hours; show understanding & tolerance to help child through this period; when possible, reorient child to name, time, place, & surrounding; know that child may also be incontinent & because of this, do not allow child to be subjected to embarrassment or disciplinary measures; explain what happened to child, parents, witnesses; speak slowly & comfortingly; check vital signs;

— teach nursing staff & family how to accurately observe & describe seizures;
— record observations in chronological sequence: time, onset of unusual behavior, environmental stimulants or other possible pre-seizure factors (photosensitivity, chill, fatigue, stressors—without interpretations or judgments), description of ictal phase, location & type of tonic or clonic contractions, presence of incontinence, skin color & condition, automisms (eye fluttering, lip smacking), eye movements & pupillary changes, duration of seizure, description of postictal phase, & progress of pt.'s condition, sensorium level of awareness, speech difficulty, weakness, pain, & length of time it takes for pt. to be reoriented & stabilized; record vital signs;
— notify MD STAT if seizures are repetitive without periods of consciousness or if seizure lasts longer than 30 minutes; know emergency protocol for status epilepticus (SE); prepare to start (& keep open) IV fluids with antiepileptic drugs (usually quick-acting diazepam to start); monitor frequently the prescribed slow infusion rate; observe closely for respiratory & cardiac depression; maintain adequate oxygenation to prevent hypoxia; suction pharynx frequently & PRN; monitor vital signs Q15 minutes & PRN; initiate I&O records; prepare to administer hypothermia measures PRN; arrange for transfer to intensive care unit or provide 1-to-1 nursing observation & care; know that EEG monitoring may be needed to differentiate SE-related from non-convulsive (stuporous) type seizures so that appropriate effective antiepileptic drug can be selected;
— after an episode of SE, observe (& take control measures) for fever, diaphoresis, hypertension; assist MD to discover SE precipitant; know that these include withdrawal from alcohol, sedatives, or antiepileptic drugs; fever, trauma, intoxication, & sleep deprivation;
— teach family that seizure threshold of child can be lowered by such factors as fatigue, sleep deprivation, infection, fever, injury, psychological stress; know that adolescents may experience a greater number of seizures before or during menstrual period & that taking diuretics sometimes helps, but should only be taken with MD approval & supervision; help family, child/youth plan a living style that manages these factors, especially stress.

2) Medication   The child will demonstrate acceptance of drug regimen by willing compliance; the child will state the importance of medication in preventing seizures; the child will help identify symptoms of side and toxic effects and will report regularly to nurse, parent, or guardian how s/he feels and when s/he notices something different:
— explain to child & family necessary information about each medication: name, dosage, time of administration, side & toxic effects to report;

- emphasize the necessity of maintaining a therapeutic blood level by not missing or postponing doses; have a clear understanding from MD what is to be done for a missed dose; explain that it may take several months to find the best combination of drugs or the most effective dosage levels;
- know that epileptics commonly feel an intense dislike for drugs that make them feel "doped up;" encourage child & family to express openly their feelings of resentment, frustration, discouragement, & skepticism; indicate that these are normal feelings that need to be recognized & ventilated;
- explain, & help child & family control, destructive behaviors (succumbing to peer pressure & social rejection by proving oneself with dangerous sports or activities, reacting to social stigma of taking daily medication by skipping doses or stopping, overprotectiveness or withdrawal from social interactions, etc.);
- have child take antiepileptic drugs with meals or large quantities of water to minimize gastric disturbances;
- know, teach, observe, record, & report promptly common side & toxic effects of antiepileptic drugs (headache, drowsiness, dizziness, rash, nausea, vomiting, gastric distress, vision disturbances, irritability, urinary frequency or retention, confusion, muscular incoordination); teach that some side effects are not obvious so periodic blood & urine tests are necessary to control seizures; it is important to teach family that close medical supervision is essential during the initial stage of determining most effective drug combinations & dosage levels;
- encourage & supervise child's practice of regular, conscientious oral hygiene; teach child & family to report any changes in gum tissue; know that oral irrigation & gum massage may slow gingival hyperplasia associated with the continued use of phenytoin (Dilantin), but because some change cannot be avoided, teach that there is a real need for regular dental evaluation & nutritional support; know that there is some evidence that phenytoin utilizes folic acid & therefore increased amounts should be added to diet; advocate softer foods for a child's tender gums.

3) Psycho-social Adjustment

The child will express his negative feelings about epilepsy and the discrimination experienced as a result; the child will accept the reality of his condition and try to live a normal life; the child will follow his medical regimen, will wear a Medic-Alert identification; the child will strive to maintain a positive self-image:

- promote & facilitate an open discussion between child, parents, teachers, & MD; bring out questions, misconceptions, fears, the reality of public discrimination, & the social stigma of epilepsy; know that child should be disciplined as a normal child, except following a seizure when behavior has not yet returned to normal;
- provide printed materials suitable for age & education; read & clarify these with pt. & family;

— encourage normal activity & exercise (activity tends to inhibit, not stimulate, seizures) but avoid excessive fatigue, chilling, overhydration, stimulation, or irregular daily schedules;

— be alert to parental behaviors that may indicate unresolved problems, e.g., overprotection, rejection of child, excessive permissiveness or punitiveness; seek mental health consultation as deemed advisable.

Discharge Planning and Teaching Objectives/Outcomes

1) (Child/Family/Guardian) Can state basic facts of epilepsy and the relevance to child's condition.
2) States s/he knows, when possible, potential stimulants to seizures and can state how they can be avoided.
3) Verbalizes knowledge of all prescribed medications (name, dosage, frequency of administration, side and toxic effects to be reported); has a written copy of this information.
4) Expresses familiarity with purpose of Epilepsy Foundation of America; has at least one of its publications and the name and address of the nearest chapter.
5) Wears a Medic-Alert (or AMA Emergency Medical) identification and carries an ID card in pocket (when appropriate for age) with information re: condition, medications, doctor name and number.
6) Has a referral to home health agency for follow-up care and information on what services are available in their community (financial help for medication and tests, special schools if needed, clinics for seizure control, etc.).

Recommended References

"Antiepileptic Drug Update: From Emergency to Maintenance," by M. Clark. *RN*, May 1980:56–63.

"Emergency Care of Seizures," by A. Williams. *Point of View* (Ethicon), July 1, 1980:10–11.

EPILEPSY: You and Your Child—A Guide for Parents, Seizure Man (comic book for children), *The Child with Epilepsy at Camp—A Guide for Counselors, School Alert Kit—A Guide for Nurse and Teacher* (for elementary or secondary level), *A Patient's Guide to EEG-Electroencephalography, Medications for Epilepsy, Role of Nurse in Epilepsy*, and other literature for parents, patients, and professionals. Landover, MD: Epilepsy Foundation of America (4351 Garden City Drive, 20785).

"Normal Growth and Development: Newborn to Adolescence." *NCP Guides #3:22–26*, 2nd Ed., Nurseco, 1983.

"Play Therapy: General Suggestions." *NCP Guide #3:30*, 2nd Ed., Nurseco, 1983.

"Psychosocial Aspects of Epilepsy," by J. Ozuna. *Journal of Neurosurgical Nursing*, December 1979:242–246.

"Screening for Seizures," by N. Santilli. *Pediatric Nursing*, March/April 1981:11–15.

"Seizure Disorders in Children: Prevention and Care," by J. Muehl. MCN: *The American Journal of Maternal Child Nursing*, May/June 1979:154–160.

"Status Epilepticus," by David Rothner and Gerald Erenburg. *Pediatric Clinics of North America*, August 1980:593–602.

"Teaching Children About Their Seizures and Medications," by M. Coughlin. MCN: *The American Journal of Maternal Child Nursing*, May/June 1979:161–162.

"The Patient with Epilepsy." *NCP Guide #3:06*, 2nd Ed., Nurseco, 1983.

"Valproic Acid for Children with Uncontrolled Epilepsy," by J. Farley. MCN: *The American Journal of Maternal Child Nursing*, May/June 1979:163–164.

The Child: Nursing Assessment Guide

A. IDENTIFICATION DATA

Name of Child/Patient (include nicknames or name familiar to child)
Sex
Age (years, months, or weeks as appropriate)
Race (ethnic origin)
Language(s) Spoken/Understood
Religious Preference

Name of Father/Guardian/Caretaker	Home Address	Telephone
Occupation	Business Address	Telephone
Name of Mother/Guardian/Caretaker	Home Address	Telephone
Occupation	Business Address	Telephone

Attending Physician
Admitting Diagnosis (if applicable or note if well-child appraisal)

B. HISTORY (identify name and age of informant; indicate opinion of reliability of information)

Present Illness (if applicable, then identify chief complaint, signs, symptoms, onset)
Current Medications, Treatments (for this as well as other conditions)
Previous Illnesses, Accidents, Injuries, Operations, Congenital Abnormalities, Developmental Disabilities
Allergies
Natal History (birth weight, length, number of weeks gestation, abnormal circumstances of labor and delivery, length of hospital stay at birth for both child and mother, neonatal period, transfusion, Rh factor, prenatal history of mother)
Developmental Growth (Denver Developmental Screening Test Results, if known and pertinent; dentition; age when first sat up alone, walked, talked; refer also to Growth and Development NCPGs #3:22–26)
Family History (significant chronic illnesses, allergies, health problems of parents, siblings, other members of household)
Living Pattern/Daily Habits
— **Nutrition:** (breast/bottle; fingers/utensils, feeds self or needs help or assistive devices; usual diet; likes and dislikes; vitamin, mineral, and fluoride supplements, quantities and eating schedule; snacking habits)

— **Elimination:** (toilet trained—urine and/or bowel movements, usual times, words used)
— **Sleep/Rest:** (quality and duration of naps/nightime sleep, usual sleeping time, routine: lights, favored objects, fluids, etc.)
— **School/Play:** (grade, performance, favorite subject, reading level, attitude toward school, attendance regularity, favorite activities, games, sports, books, toys, TV shows, playmates, pets, hobbies)
— **Social/Emotional Behavior:** (relationship with siblings, sitters and caretakers, other household adults; personality characteristics: introvert/extrovert, dependent/independent, timid, shy, aggressive, etc.; tensional outlets and mannerisms such as nail biting, hair twisting, rocking, crying, etc.; usual coping mechanisms such as talkativeness, inquisitiveness, joking, laughter, imaginary playmates or pets; typical reactions to new situations or to previously stressful situations; phobias of sudden onset, fear of strangers/men/darkness/ being alone; signs of social withdrawal, depression, hostility, aggression; history of declining school performance, running away from home, age-inappropriate sex play, excessive or public masturbation)
— **Environmental Factors:** (location of home, population density, sanitary conditions, proximity to pollutants: air, water, dust, lead paint/pipes/dishes, asbestos, chemicals, aerosol can usage, smoking members of household; accessibility of medications, drugs, alcohol, insecticides, cleaning products, garage chemicals, firearms, home or neighborhood violence, poisonous house or yard plants)
— **Cultural/Religious/Socio-Economic Background:** (problems in understanding English, non-English speaking or limited English proficiency; factors related to step-parents, half-siblings, custody issues, non-related adults in household income, employment, and ability to pay for needed food, medications, transportation, & treatment)

C. **PHYSICAL EXAMINATION** (refer to NCPGs #4:47–50, "Physical Assessment, Parts A, B, C, D")
Vital Signs (TPR and BP: site taken, rate, and quality; note presence of stridor, retractions, cough, irregularities)
Body Measurements (height, weight, size, contour of head, fontanels, chest, and abdomen)
General Appearance (description of coloring, state of nutrition and development, features)
Neurological System (sensorium: alert, semi-comatose, responsive to verbal and/or painful stimuli; irritable, crying, seizures, tremors, paralysis, weakness: type, description, location, reflexes)
Status of Skin, Hair, Scalp, and Appendages (color, condition: temperature, moisture, edema, identifying marks, bruises, rashes, abrasions; scars: location, description)

Status of Special Senses
— **Eyes/Vision:** (color and condition of sclera, iris, conjunctiva, eyelids; glasses, contact lenses, strabismus, twitching)
— **Ears/Hearing:** (symmetry, placement, ability to hear tuning forks, soft voice, hearing aids)
— **Nose/Smelling:** (discharge, bleeding, deviated septum, patency of nostrils)
— **Throat/Taste/Speech/Mouth/Teeth:** (abnormal lip or palate; broken, missing, or crooked teeth; color and condition of mouth/gums/throat; difficulty sucking, swallowing, speaking)

Gastrointestinal System (nausea/vomiting, hematemesis, constipation/diarrhea, last meal taken when)

Genitourinary System (characteristics of urine and urinary pattern, incontinence, enuresis, structure of genitals; note circumcision, examine for descended testicles)

Musculoskeletal System (condition and mobility of neck, back, arms, legs; note braces, contractures, finger clubbing, clubbing, evidence of old fractures, deformities; evaluate for scoliosis, uneven leg length, posture, walking)

D. RELEVANT NEEDS/PROBLEMS/CONCERNS OF PARENT/GUARDIAN/CARETAKER

Status of Understanding (what does s/he know? what does s/he need to know re: diagnosis? treatment? prognosis? care? child's level of bio/psycho/social development?)

Parent-Child Relationship (verbal communications, feeling tones, body language, touch and warmth of interactions)

Level of Desired Involvement (indicative of parents' feelings/attitudes about child's care and how much reponsibility and participation they wish to have; understanding and acceptance of parental role with its incumbent adaptations and sacrifices)

Recommended References
"A Developmental Approach to Physical Assessment," by L. Yoos. *MCN: American Journal of Maternal Child Nursing*, May/June 1981:168–170.
"Helping Young People Cope with the Physical Examination," by J.R. Moss. *Pediatric Nursing*, March/April 1981:17–20.
"Normal Growth & Development: Newborn to Adolescent." *NCP Guides #3:22–26*, 2nd Ed., Nurseco, 1983.
"Physical Assessment: Parts A, B, C, and D." *NCP Guides #4:47–50*, 2nd Ed., Nurseco, 1983.
"Symposium on Child Abuse and Neglect. Sexual Abuse of Children: Case Finding and Clinical Assessment," by J. Thomas and C. Rogers. *Nursing Clinics of North America*, March 1981:179–188.

The Child Experiencing Separation Anxiety

Definition: Separation anxiety is an anticipation of danger or uncertainty rather than a direct reaction to danger. It is the result of stress that is generated by separating a child from his significant others, usually parents.

LONG TERM GOAL: The child will experience this period of separation with minimal traumatic and/or residual effects, and will integrate separation experiences into his concepts of security and trust for others.

General Considerations:
— Separation anxiety is related to a child's pursuit of security and identity. The *behaviors* that accompany it can be divided into three recognizable stages or phases: protest, despair, and detachment or denial.
— **Some stress is essential** to normal psychological growth; the right amount at the right time stimulates the maturation of the child; stress becomes overwhelming for any one child if the adaptive capacity of that child and the support systems available to him are inadequate.
— **Learning to separate from parents** is normally a gradual process achieved by the child as s/he comes to appreciate his separate individuality; it cannot be forced abruptly.
— **The separation involved in hospitalization,** coupled with the stress of illness, is *usually beyond* the normal adaptive capacity of a young child (eight months to six years).
— **Children with the greatest risk** for experiencing moderate to high levels of separation anxiety are those under six years of age, only or youngest children, ones who have had limited contacts outside the home, and children who have recently experienced a traumatic separation.
— **Nursing responsibilities** include assessing the stage and degree of separation anxiety, assisting the child and parent/guardian to cope with the anxiety in a productive, effective manner, and supporting hospital policies that promote increased interaction, visiting hours, and parenting roles of parents or caretakers. Nurses should incorporate into the written care plan findings of the nursing history regarding the child's previous activities: time of awakening, feeding times and methods, likes and dislikes, play patterns and toys, naptime and bedtime rituals, and other significant behavior patterns, so they can be promoted during hospitalization as much as possible.
— Review NCPGs #3:22–26, "Normal Growth & Development," for appropriate age level.

Specific Considerations, Potential Patient Outcomes, and Nursing Actions:

1) Stage of Protest

The child will experience minimal effect of loss of parent; the child will not injure self or others; the child will maintain a secure and trusting relationship with parent(s); the child will accept care of nursing staff:

— know that the stage of protest begins with hospitalization or mother's absence & lasts from a few hours to 3 or 4 days; know that the common behaviors of this stage include:
  - restlessness & crying
  - crying out for mother, demanding her presence
  - listening for her step & looking for her to come
  - intensified crying when parents leave & when demands are not met
  - puffy eyes, red face
  - refusal to go to sleep
  - refusal to cooperate with care or treatment procedures
  - fighting, struggling, resisting, or pushing caretakers away;

— be accepting of crying & anger; reassure child that mother will be back, using language appropriate for age & stage of development;

— delay intrusive procedures when child is most upset;

— stay visible but do not force contact with child; respond to the child physically when s/he initiates contact, then cuddle & comfort ad lib;

— gently restrain child if s/he attempts to escape or injure self or others; use crib nets or jacket restraints PRN;

— provide child with familiar & cherished objects, if possible;

— encourage parents to visit as often as able; explain child's behavior to them;

— be warm, firm, & reassuring to child;

— allow for safe areas like crib, playroom;

— read to child *Curious George Goes to the Hospital*;

— use puppets, comedy to attract child's attention & cooperation;

— consider visiting child's home prior to admission to alleviate fears & reduce incidence of hospitalization anxiety, or arrange for child to visit hospital (tour & pre-admission party);

— if the child has had an emergency admission, & if the child is placed in a Pediatric Intensive Care Unit (PICU), know that both child & family will encounter a varying combination of additional stressors, such as:
- nature & severity of child's illness
- restrictions & fright caused by necessary treatment (restraints, intrusive procedures, machines)
- sleep deprivation
- unfamiliar surroundings compounded by altered states of consciousness related to disease, fever, & drugs
- imposed separation of family related to space limitations or the emotional impact of critically ill child on the parent (e.g., grief, shock, guilt, etc.)
- sensory stimuli (e.g., noxious odors)
- imposed bed rest
- threat to child's body image, integrity, control of functions, as well as pain or fear of pain;

— assess the actual effects of PICU stressors & plan care according to individual needs of child & family; provide PRN additional explanations, encouragement, touching/stroking, talking/soothing, environmental manipulation to reduce stressors, allowing the child to make some simple decisions.

2) Stage of Despair

The child will demonstrate understanding and acceptance of separation by cheerfulness, cooperation, and participation in play activities in order to express and to cope more effectively with feelings:

— know that the stage of despair is frequently called the mourning state or "settling in" stage, & lasts 1-2 days or may persist until discharge; know that the common behaviors of this stage include:
- regressive behavior such as thumbsucking, holding blanket or toy, soiling bed with feces, incontinence, whining, clinging, or use of baby talk
- apathy & withdrawal; sometimes hyperactive or overtly aggressive
- staying in crib in a fetal position, pretending to be asleep
- happy to see parent, but crying with protest when parent leaves
- demanding to be taken home
- accepting nursing care passively
- allowing staff to handle & touch him/her;

— allow regressive behavior, but do not foster or encourage it;
— do not put on diapers automatically or give all children a bottle; rather, do a careful admission assessment to determine normal behavior patterns;
— provide for physical comfort & closeness; hold & rock child, establish trust;
— attempt to maintain skills achieved at home like talking, potty training; know that the last skill learned will be the first to disappear;
— allow expression of anger through play with active toys like play clay, bang toys, balls, or dramatic play with puppets, dolls; refer to NCPG #3:30, "Play Therapy;"
— use games like peek-a-boo or hide-and-seek to desensitize child to separation; tell stories where people are reunited or together;
— keep track of child's possessions & do not lose them; allow child to wear own clothes; have shoes at bedside as knows s/he will need them to go home;
— have mother leave something of hers behind, like a purse or gloves, so child knows she will return for them & him; have bedside pictures of family, pet, or best friend; continue to explain child's behavior to parent & encourage parent to verbalize feelings of confusion, sadness, anxiety, etc.;
— whenever possible, enable parents to participate actively in the care and comfort of child.

3) Stage of Denial or Detachment

The child will maintain socially effective defense mechanisms; the child will interact normally and effectively with peers and adults:
— know that the stage of denial or detachment is a period of acceptance or adjustment with a return to normal patterns of behavior, but this may not be achieved before discharge if hospitalization is 4 days or less, or if the child is in a PICU; know that the common behaviors of this stage include:
  • showing an interest in surroundings & others
  • accepting care & love from almost anyone
  • complacency
  • no acting-out behavior or frequent bursts of anger
  • playing well by self or with others
  • greets parents happily or may ignore their presence; when parents leave, may cry only for a few minutes & then is easily distracted to another activity;

- continue previous nursing actions that have been successful;
- encourage expression of fears in play;
- talk about home, what the people are doing there now, about when s/he will be going home to room/school/brother/sister, & what s/he will do;
- continue use of physical contact;
- explain to parents child's need to be held even if it appears that s/he rejects them;
- help parents continue role (they tend to resent nurses' acceptance by child & feel they are stealing child's love); if parents pull back now, child will *know* s/he is being abandoned as s/he has suspected;
- allow child to have some control over his life & the things that are done to him; let him be involved with other children.

Recommended References

"Are Hospitalized Toddlers Adapting to the Experience as Well as We Think?" by J. Calkin. *MCN: American Journal of Maternal Child Nursing*, January/February 1979:18–23.
"Books for the Hospitalized Child," by A. Galligan. *American Journal of Nursing*, December 1975:2164–2166.
Curious George Goes to the Hospital, by M. and H.S. Rey. Boston: Houghton Mifflin, 1966.
"How Can You Improve Care of the Hospitalized Child? . . . This Assessment Tool Can Help," by J. Meissner. *Nursing 80*, October 1980:50–51.
"Humanistic Nursing Care for Critically Ill Children," by K. Stevens. *Nursing Clinics of North America*, December 1981:611–622.
"Normal Growth and Development: Newborn to Adolescent." *NCP Guides #3:22–26*, 2nd Ed., Nurseco, 1983.
"Nursing Aspects of Pediatric Intensive Care in a General Hospital," by M. Soupios et al. *Pediatric Clinics of North America*, August 1980:621–632.
"Play Therapy: General Suggestions." *NCP Guide #3:30*, 2nd Ed., Nurseco, 1983.
"Using Roy's Concept of Adaptation to Care for Young Children," by A. Galligan. *MCN: American Journal of Maternal Nursing*, January/February 1979:24–28.

The Child with a Tonsillectomy and Adenoidectomy (T&A)

Definition: Tonsillectomy is the surgical excision of both tonsils; adenoidectomy is the surgical excision of adenoid tissue. Adenotonsillectomy is the combined operative procedure.

LONG TERM GOAL: The child will return to his home and family following safe, successful surgery; the child will integrate this experience into his self-concept; the child will maintain the ongoing processes of growth and development and will resume his normal life functioning within the family.

General Considerations:

— **Incidence:** still widely common, nevertheless significantly decreased with the advent of antibiotics and the growth in medical and legal controversy over the advisability of the operation.

— The tonsils are a major factor in the early immunity defensive structures used by the body to decrease the incidence and spread of respiratory and other infections. They should only be removed after the considered evaluation by the physician that the harm of remaining tonsils outweighs their protective function.

— The tonsils are usually larger during the infant and toddler years and then become smaller as the child reaches school age. Surgery during this pre-school period should be postponed, and the child with frequent sore throats treated with antibiotics. In addition, the emotional and psychological effects of surgery during the pre-school period are more traumatic than when the child is much older.

— **Indications for a tonsillectomy** are: (1) marked hypertrophy of tonsils causing airway obstruction, distorted speech, swallowing difficulties with subsequent nutrition-related weight loss, marked hypertension, or cor pulmonale; (2) tonsillar malignancy; (3) diphtheria carrier; and (4) repeated severe, laboratory-documented streptococcal infections (more than seven bouts in one year or three to five episodes in two or more successive years).

— An **adenoidectomy** is a separate operation carrying specific and separate indications: (1) marked hypertrophy causing hypoxia, cor pulmonale, severe speech distortion, or dental and facial abnormalities, or (2) when associated with chronic otitis media and its complications of hearing loss or mastoiditis. Present conservative treatment of acute otitis media advocates antibiotics, a myringotomy, and a tympanostomy tube.

— Although T&A or adenotonsillectomy is often thought of and carried out as a single combined operation, each should be considered separately regarding its risks and benefits. In any case, neither operation should be performed on children with blood dyscrasias, leukemia, or bleeding disorders.

— **Nursing responsibilities** include assessment of the child's normal growth and development, his/her age-appropriate adaptation to the experience of hospitalization and surgery, pre- and postoperative intervention individualized to minimize apprehension and complications and to maximize energy available for the healing process, and education of the child and parents according to response and need.

Specific Considerations, Potential Patient Outcomes, and Nursing Actions:

1) Apprehension and Fear

The child will feel less apprehensive and fearful; the child will receive pre-op teaching according to maturational ability:
— refer to NCPGs #3:22–26, "Normal Growth & Development," for appropriate age level;
— assist parents with pre-op teaching by supplying facts, simulated equipment, & a pre-hospitalization tour;
— allow child to handle equipment prior to its use; provide honest, simple, & direct answers to his questions;
— encourage parents to stay with pt., to tell him when they leave, & when they are coming back;
— observe child's reactions in play situations & listen to what s/he tells you—offer supportive reassurance;
— read to the child the book, *Madeline* (if age appropriate, under 10);
— refer to NCPG #3:20, "The Child Experiencing Separation Anxiety," for additional information & nursing actions.

2) Prevention of Complications

The child will have a stable post-op condition with bleeding controlled; the child will be free of preventable complications or, if occurring, will have them promptly detected and optimally managed:
— monitor pulse & respirations (rate & quality) at least Q2H for signs of increasing frequency that reflect bleeding; observe for hypotension, checking BP regularly as ordered until stable;
— record & monitor carefully rectal temp Q2H; notify MD & document all temps of 38.3°C (101°F) lasting more than 12 hours, or a single spike greater than 38.9°C (102°F);
— observe & report respiratory distress, "crowing," retraction of chest muscles;
— inspect throat, observe frequency of swallowing & note any vomiting as these symptoms may indicate hemorrhage (chances of bleeding are highest in the 1st 48 hours & again between the 7th & 10th PO day);
— chart accurate I&O; record urine specific gravity at least Q4H;
— avoid use of aspirin for pain as it increases possibility of bleeding;
— administer antibiotics prophylactically as ordered.

3) Rest and Comfort	The patient will experience moderate comfort, will be able to breathe easily without danger of aspirating secretions:

— provide a side-lying position without a pillow;
— remind pt. to avoid coughing or clearing throat as much as possible; have pt. gently spit up mucus or bloody drainage; record presence or absence of tonsillar packing;
— give mouth care; rinse with cold water Q1–2H & ad lib;
— apply ice collar to reduce discomfort, swelling, & likelihood of bleeding; change as necessary to keep cold;
— offer ice chips or popsicles when pt. is fully alert & nausea has subsided; milkshakes, ice cream, & mild juices are often given the evening of surgical day as both the softness & coldness of these products help to reduce swelling & diminish soreness;
— turn & deep breathe Q2H;
— maintain bed rest with BRP in a quiet environment to encourage rest; check for pain, restlessness, bleeding at least Q2H during 1st post-op night.

Discharge Planning and Teaching Objectives/Outcomes:

1) (Parent/Guardian) Verbalizes knowledge to keep child quiet for a few days, to continue soft foods and fluids, and to protect child from contact with infection, especially URI.
2) Verbalizes realization that symptoms like earache, persistent coughing, swallowing, or vomiting of blood require a physician's attention.
3) Can identify medications ordered, state their correct usage, and tell why it is important to avoid medications that contain aspirin.
4) Can state date and time of follow-up medical appointment.

Recommended References

"Layman's Guide to Common Complaints. Part 8 Tonsillitis," by I. Librach. *Nursing Mirror*, September 13, 1979:18–19.
Madeline, by L. Bemelmans. New York: Viking, 1967.
"Normal Growth and Development: Newborn to Adolescent." *NCP Guides #3:22–26*, 2nd Ed., Nurseco, 1983.
"T & A Controversy—When Should Tonsils and/or Adenoids Go?" by A. Brodoff. *Patient Care*, November 30, 1979:116–117.
"The Child Experiencing Separation Anxiety." *NCP Guide #3:20*, 2nd Ed., Nurseco, 1983.
"Tonsillectomy and Adenoidectomy," by J. Paradise. *Pediatric Clinics of North America*, November 1981:881–891.

Normal Growth and Development: Neonate

Definition: Growth is a measurable increase in physical size of the whole or any of its parts. Development is a dynamic process of change following a sequential pattern resulting in a progressive increase in ability and potential. Neonate is the period of an infant's life from birth to one month.

LONG TERM GOAL: The newborn will achieve the highest level of potential growth and development; the infant with developmental disabilities will have them correctly identified early in life and have special needs met to facilitate maximum development.

General Considerations:
— **A child's growth follows an orderly, predictable pattern** from general to specific, from head to foot (cephalocaudal), from center to periphery (proximodistal), and from simple to complex (e.g., gross to fine motor development). Rate and focus of growth and development shifts or fluctuates (spurts and dormant periods) during successive periods.
— **Similar patterns** of growth and development exist between children, but patterns are statistical averages, *not* absolute standards for any one child to meet. Since any child's genetic potential for growth can be influenced by environmental factors such as nutrition, climate, exercise, and socioeconomic status of the family, one must accept the absolute uniqueness of each child.
— **The first month** of a newborn's life is a crucial period of great adaptation and rapid growth and development. The newborn needs to adjust to other people, to establish a relationship with a consistent, loving caregiver (usually mother), and to perform adequately the normal physiological functions of eating, sleeping, responding to stimulation, and adapting to the environment. Long-term bio/psycho/social/emotional and cognitive development are affected by the kind of start a baby gets in life.
— **ANA Maternal-Child Health Standard #2:** "Maternal and child health nursing practice is based upon knowledge of the biophysical and psychosocial development of individuals from conception through the child-rearing phase of development and upon knowledge of the basic needs for optimum development."
— **Nursing responsibilities** include being knowledgeable about normal patterns of both physical and psychosocial growth and development; identifying patterns that represent growth and utilizing these patterns and their implications as a guide for assessing the neonate; helping parents understand the changes inherent with this growth process; and assisting the infant to attain the highest possible level of development. Studies show that mothers with early performance expectations provide more stimulating home environments and the infants have higher scores on developmental tests, compared to mothers who have lower, later developmental expectations. The latter group are also likely to be poorer, have less education, and have fewer psychosocial assets to

draw upon (e.g., less emotional support from significant others; some negative feelings about pregnancy, labor, and delivery; low self-esteem and self-confidence, etc.). Appropriate expectations and parenting skills do not come naturally. They must be learned, and therefore should be taught by child health specialists, in the hospital, in the clinic, and in the home so that parents can more successfully encourage optimum development.

— **The common parameters** of physical development and behaviors for the neonate are outlined below, together with corresponding nursing implications and teaching or guidance suggestions. Succeeding NCPGs (#3:23–26) cover the periods from infancy through adolescence.

Neonate: Birth to 1 month

Physical Development

— **Weight:** 2500–3850 gms (5.5–8 lbs) average; initially loses 5–12 oz (5–10%) of birth weight; average weight gain during 10th to 30th day of life is 1 oz/day.

— **Height:** 47.5–53.75 cm (19–21") average

— **Heart Rate:** 120–160 beats/minute
— **Pulses Present:** femoral & dorsalis pedis

— **Respirations:** 30–60/minute; diaphragmatic & abdominal breathing; bilateral breath sounds

Nursing Implications

— Weigh neonates nude on the same scale at the same time daily before a feeding; report any weight loss or failure to gain weight after hospital discharge to the physician. Breastfed babies may take 10–14 days to recover their birth weight. Community health nurse referral is advocated for any newborns with low birth weight, anticipated feeding problems, or weight progression problems.

— Heart rate & respirations are frequently irregular in neonates. Vital signs require careful monitoring for signs of infection, dehydration, & hypoglycemia. Accurate blood pressure monitoring requires special sized equipment, special norms table.

— Monitor & evaluate increasing respiratory rate, since newborns increase own body temperature by increasing respirations.
— Suction nose with bulb syringe prior to feeding if there is congestion or mucus. Always suction mouth first because neonate is an obligatory nose breather. Provide postural drainage to clear tract. Newborns cannot cough up secretions.

Physical Development

— **Temperature:** irregular for first 8–12 hours; averages 37.2°C (99°F) rectally, depending on clothing & environmental temperature.

— **Hemoglobin:** 18–20 gm

— **Head Circumference:** 34–35 cm (13–14''); equals or exceeds chest circumference. Diamond-shaped anterior fontanel open (covered with tough membrane) about 2.5–4 cm in width; soft & flat to touch. Posterior fontanel may be closed.

— **Chest:** 30.5–33 cm (12–13'')

— **Skin:** dry, turgor is firm, elastic; physiologic jaundice in a normal term infant appears after 24 hours & disappears by 7th day. Milia (tiny cysts of obstructed sebaceous glands) appear on face, especially across bridge of nose; disappear without treatment. Toxic erythema (papules lasting 2 or 3 days) may appear first 2 weeks of life in 30–70% of normal infants; also disappears without treatment. Mongolian spots on black infants, often around buttocks, disappear spontaneously in a few weeks or months.

Nursing Implications

— Use rectal thermometer; lubricate, insert gently just past anal sphincter.
— Newborn skin is thin & capillaries do not contract adequately to maintain body heat. Dress newborn according to environmental need for warmth, but prevent overheating because neonates do not sweat to lower body heat. Teach parents these facts, since overdressing & underdressing are common.

— Head circumference & fontanel status are primary indicators of changes in intracranial pressure; observations by the same individual at regular intervals are desirable; an increase of greater than 0.5 cm per week requires further evaluation. Depressed anterior fontanel may indicate dehydration.

— Teach mother normal bathing procedures with mild, nonmedicated soap. Explain common skin lesions & assure that they will disappear without special treatment. Tell mothers to report all rashes & lesions that do not disappear in a few days.
— Some babies do not lose cord before end of 3 weeks. Tell mother to keep cord dry & exposed to air until it falls off & to avoid tub baths during this time.

Physical Development

— **Muscles:** muscle tone strong & equal bilaterally when extending extremities; posture & movement symmetrical. Gluteal folds are usually symmetrical; asymmetry may or may not be pathologically significant. Tremors are brief, spontaneous, rhythmic, & common in neonates.

— **Genitalia:** swollen vagina, labia; vaginal discharge (mucus, sometimes blood-tinged) 1st week; swollen scrotum, descended testicles

— **Stools:** meconium, greenish-black first 2–4 days; transition from greenish-brown to yellow; if breastfed, may have from 0–6 stools/24 hours, golden mustard & unformed; if bottle-fed, stools will be light yellow, more formed, & more frequent than those of a breastfed newborn.

— **Immune System:** the neonate possesses a passive immunity from mother that protects from some illnesses. Even so, the immune system is immature & newborns are vulnerable to sudden, severe illness.

Common Behaviors

— **Movements:** reflexive, random, uncoordinated; head sags when unsupported, but control is more effective than once thought; neck, arm, & shoulder muscles contract to help newborn assume an upright position. (Hypotonic or hypoxic neonates have little or no head control & neck is extremely lax.)

Nursing Implications

— Failure of legs to abduct 180° can be indicative of congenital hip dislocation; x-rays are often indicated for further evaluation.

— Distinguishing tremors or jitteriness from seizure activity is important. Careful observation & precise recording is essential. Note abnormal eye movements, blinking eyes, circumoral cyanosis, sucking or chewing movements, periods of apnea, changed cry or behavior.

— Teach mother that newborn may go a day or 2 without stools, if breastfed, & that very soft stools are common, they are not diarrhea.

— Parents should be urged to keep baby away from large groups of people, especially for 1st month. Parents need to be taught to observe & report immediately signs of illness (fever, weight loss, poor feeding, vomiting, diarrhea, excessive irritability & crying, lethargy, respiratory distress).

Parental Guidance Suggestions

— Safety measures for holding, supporting head, handling, & diapering cannot be overemphasized. Review at every parental contact, taking care to point out the developmental changes of the baby & its growing abilities.

Common Behaviors

— **Reflexes:** should be strong, immediate, coordinated; unique to the first weeks & months of life; they include *sucking & rooting* (lst year), *palmar grasp* (disappears in 4–6 months), *plantar grasp* (lasts 8–15 months), *tonic neck reflex* (first 6 months), *stepping or dance reflex* (six weeks), *Moro or startle reflex* (fades 1–4 months), *swallowing & coughing* (persists & strengthens).

— **Vocalization:** makes throaty noises; crying is vigorous, involves the total body & is the primary method of making needs known. Periodic bouts of loud, irritable crying are common. "Colic" crying occurs with expulsion of flatus, starts & stops suddenly for no apparent reason or attempt to comfort; usually stops entirely by 3rd or 4th month.

— **Visual:** newborn has limited depth perception; sees objects approximately 8–12" away; follows voices & objects, showing special interest in human faces; sensitive to bright lights, will close eyes; gazes longer at patterns & figures than at plain designs; seems to prefer red & yellow colors; eyes are small & functionally immature; eye movements are not yet coordinated.

Parental Guidance Suggestions

— Teach parents to identify newborn needs for crying (hunger, wetness, loud noises, strong odors, wish to be held) & to meet needs satisfactorily; to report to nurse or doctor excessive crying (more than 2 hours in 24).

— Burp, rock, & sing to baby; try playing soft music near baby's crib; give pacifier to meet baby's needs for more sucking time than feedings allow.

— Show objects & smiling, friendly faces to newborns at a distance of 12" when possible; hang bed mobiles 7–9" from baby's eyes; use homemade mobiles made with bright, colorful objects rather than some commercial mobiles that are uninteresting when viewed from the bottom upwards.

— If tear duct is blocked, baby's eye will not drain tears properly and cannot blink correctly to avoid dust particles, increasing the risk of infection. Consult MD; rinse eye with sterile water & massage inner canthus gently twice daily for a week or so until blockage disappears. (MD may want to open tear duct in office with a simple procedure.)

Common Behaviors

— **Auditory:** attends to voices, turning head to follow; affected by sound frequency; attention more often attracted by female voices & by higher pitched, falsetto-type voices; loud noises lead to startle reflex.

— **Taste:** can discriminate between sweet & non-sweet; newborns, especially girls, prefer sweet taste.

— **Smell:** discriminates between odors; strong odors that adults find annoying cause babies to cry, turn head away, & become active. May sneeze or sniffle because nasal hairs are not developed enough to clear nasal passages of mucus.

— **Touch:** sensitive to touch; has a strong need for tactile stimulation all over body; keeps hands fisted & drops objects placed in hands.

— **Sleep:** 20–22 hours

Parental Guidance Suggestions

— Talk to baby often; play soft music or have a ticking clock nearby; expose to normal household sounds, but protect from unduly loud noises.

— Sweetened water is useful to encourage intake of water, but avoid letting infant get accustomed to over-sweetened fluids.

— Protect newborn from strong odors.
— Gently clean mucus from end of nose with a damp wash cloth; apply a small dab of petroleum jelly near the nasal openings (not inside) to prevent irritations & crusting of mucus.

— Hold newborn, rock, cuddle, pat, caress, touch, & stroke when awake; play with baby; keep infant nearby as much as possible so it is convenient to touch often; swaddle in soft clothing & blankets, varying positions from time to time when awake or when sleeping. Tell parents that infant carriers made of cloth held next to the parent's body help meet the tactile needs of child; teach them to assure head support when carrying like this.

— Allow newborn to sleep as desired, at least 2–3 hours between feedings.

Common Behaviors
— **Feeding:** feeds from bottle or breast; occasionally CNS or congenitally damaged neonates may require gavage or gastrostomy feedings. Requires 16–24 oz fluid/day for adequate weight gain (commercial formulas & breast milk contain approximately 20 calories/ounce). Average gain during 10th to 30th day of life is approximately 1 oz/day.

Parental Guidance Suggestions
— Newborn's rapid metabolic rate predisposes neonate to fluid & electrolyte imbalance & hypoglycemia. The stomach empties in 2–4 hours. Breastfeeders often require feeding Q2H; formula intake should average 2½ oz/lb/day. Supplement formula with water bottle to insure adequate fluid intake. Generally use iron-supplemented formula.
— Hold infant for all feedings. Let neonate set the pace of feeding. Be sure nipple provides a slow, steady stream of milk when newborn sucks; burp after every ounce taken (some babies won't allow this interruption). Place infant on side or abdomen with head turned to side after feeding to prevent aspiration of regurgitations. Mild regurgitation is common due to swallowed air & temporary incompetence of cardiac sphincter. Vomiting of any kind should be immediately reported to doctor, especially if it occurs more than once.
— Assess maternal-newborn interaction during feeding; help mother to interpret newborn's cues & achieve success in feeding; reinforce mother's optimism, positive feelings about self & nurturing behavior; know that mothers feel guilty & inadequate when newborn fails to feed satisfactorily, even though it may not be their fault. Refer PRN to NCPGs #4:30, "The Mother Who Breastfeeds Her Infant," & #4:32, "Parent-Infant Bonding."

Recommended References

"Assessment as a Method of Enhancing Infant Development," by T. B. Brazelton, MD. *Zero to Three* (Bulletin of the National Center for Clinical Infant Programs), September 1981.

"The First Year: The First Week," "The First Month." *American Baby*, Mid-February 1981:12–35.

"The Mother Who Breastfeeds Her Infant." *NCP Guide #4:30*, 2nd Ed., Nurseco, 1983.

Newborn Family and Nurse, 2nd Ed., by M. Moore. Philadelphia: Saunders,1981.

"Newborn Feeding Behaviors and Attaching," by L. Taylor. *MCN: The American Journal of Maternal Child Nursing*, May/June 1981:210–202.

"New Findings about Mother's Antenatal Expectations and Their Relationship to Infant Development," by C. Snyder et al. *MCN: The American Journal of Maternal Child Nursing*, November/December 1979:354–358.

"Parent-Infant Bonding." *NCP Guide #4:32*, 2nd Ed., Nurseco, 1983.

Standards of Maternal-Child Health Nursing Practice. Kansas City, MO: American Nurses Association, 1973.

Normal Growth & Development: Infant

Definition: The initial period of an individual baby's life cycle, generally spanning from four weeks to eighteen months.

LONG TERM GOAL: The infant will develop to its fullest genetic potential, proceeding toward maturity with optimum health, well-being, and a sense of trust in care-givers or primary nurturers.

General Considerations:
— Refer to NCPG #3:22, "Normal Growth & Development: Neonate."
— Childhood is sequentially divided into stages or critical periods to denote a specific span of time that is maximally favorable for the accomplishment of a new developmental process or task.
— **Developmental task** (Erikson's central problem) to be resolved in infancy is the development of a sense of *trust* versus *mistrust*.
— Overall **nursing responsibilities** during infancy include meeting the infant's needs for nutrition, warmth, sucking, comfort, sensory stimulation, security, and love; supporting and guiding the parents to a responsible, nurturing, and understanding relationship with their child; observing, assessing, and recording normal and abnormal patterns of infant growth and development; and becoming more aware of own attitudes, beliefs, values, and feelings regarding child rearing practices as well as the wide range of ethnic and cultural diversity in family backgrounds.
— The **common parameters** of physical development and behaviors for the infant are outlined below, together with corresponding nursing implications and teaching or guidance suggestions.

One to Six Months

Physical Development
— **Weight:** gains 5–8 oz/week. Average American baby now doubles birth weight by 4⅔ months.
— **Height:** grows approximately 1"/month.

— **Posterior Fontanel:** closes about 2 months.

— **Teething:** begins approximately 5–6 months; drools excessively as unable to swallow saliva.

Nursing Implications and Parental Guidance Suggestions
— Review with parents the accuracy of their knowledge on formula or breastfeeding techniques.
— Teach normal growth & development & safety needs to parents, repeating PRN.
— While fontanels remain open, show parents how to handle head gently, but not be afraid to wash scalp.
— Suggest a bib to absorb saliva.

Physical Development

— **Reflexes:** sucks reflexively in response to touch; quiets in response to sucking.
- strong palmar grasp reflex; reaches to mouth; "mouths" objects and fist at two months; chews at 4–6 months.
- Moro (startle) reflex present from birth to 4 months.
- tonic neck reflex response reaches peak about 3 months, then gradually disappears.

— **Skin:** diaper rashes common; red rash around face at about 4–5 weeks is common; lasts 4–6 weeks, disappears without treatment; is thought to be associated with disappearance of mother's hormones & the activation of baby's oil & sweat glands.

— **Immunity:** passive immunity received from mother is lost unless infant is breastfeeding; then immunity to some diseases remains through breastfeeding period.

Nursing Implications and Parental Guidance Suggestions

— Encourage parents to use a pacifier or let baby suck its fingers or thumb, since sucking needs are often stronger than feeding time satisfies.

— Warn parents to be sure that all objects within baby's reach are too large to be swallowed; provide washable, safe toys.

— Try to avoid loud noises or startling moves around baby.

— Since baby exhibits a definite preference for turning head to one side, tell parents to turn baby's head periodically to prevent unsightly flattening of head from sleeping too much with head turned to preferred side. Suggest reversing crib's position in room or hanging bright objects on the neglected side of the crib to stimulate interest.

— Remind parent to keep diaper area clean & dry; protect skin with thin layer of water-barrier ointment (zinc ointment, petroleum jelly, hydrogenated vegetable shortening); avoid perfumed soaps & any bubble bath products.

— Encourage parents to seek medical care at physician's recommended intervals, usually 6 weeks, 3, 6, 9, 12, & 18 months. Ascertain that parents have a doctor who is available, accessible, & within transportation & financial means. Assess parents' feelings of confidence in selves & in their doctor. Make sure they have phone number of someone who may be called for simple, sympathetic guidance, & also for an emergency accident or illness.

— Assure parents of need to have immunizations at recommended visits, beginning with DPT & TOPV (Trivalent Oral Polio Vaccine).

Physical Development

Common Behaviors
Two months
— **Movement:** can move in crib; holds head erect in mid position for a few seconds, but still wobbly.

— **Play:** likes bright, colorful, large toys of varied shapes, configurations, & textures; spongy, squeezable toys that make sounds.

Nursing Implications and Parental Guidance Suggestions
— Provide immunization record for parent to keep.
— Explain possible side effects of immunization (fever, irritability, fussiness) & what to do (possibly liquid antipyretic or tepid bath).
— Immunization with DPT is now not recommended for infants with a family history of CNS disorders.
— Review common signs of illness & importance of early medical attention.

Parental Guidance Suggestions

— Be certain crib slats are no greater than 2¼" apart.
— Secure infant seat so it cannot tip over with baby's movement.
— Use only safety approved carseats that meet new Federal standards.
— Encourage parents to find out about Red Cross Baby Care Classes in their community.
— Toys should be washable & durable without sharp edges or small, loose pieces; avoid fuzzy toys (present an inhalation danger).
— Use crib gyms with items for grabbing; rotate toys in crib or playpen to provide various stimuli.
— Use infant seats & swings for awake baby. Sometimes place baby in prone position with toys around him; other times, use back or chest carrier to keep baby close to mother. Avoid excessive use of infant seat.

Common Behaviors

— **Crying:** becomes differentiated as to cause, i.e., pain, cold, offensive odors, loud noises.
— **Smile:** an open-eyed, alert smile involving whole face, eyes crinkling; responds to another's smile.
— **Vision:** can follow a bright, moving object or from outer corner of eye to midline; stares indefinitely at surroundings, fixating on 1 or 2 objects (especially moving objects); prefers person to object; begins to coordinate senses (i.e., sucking at sight of bottle, anticipating or looking for sound of objects); attempts to bat or grab objects; begins to hold objects for a few moments.
— **Sleep:** 18–20 hours/day; may sleep 7 hours at night after a late night feeding; shows a definite preference for sleep position; stays awake longer when people interact with him/her.
— **Feeding:** needs approximately 115 calories/kg/day; eats approximately Q4H & anticipates feedings. Breastfeeders may eat more frequently if the mother's milk supply is not adequate to meet the baby's needs.
— **Bathing:** enjoys bath, kicking, & splashing; exhibits delight & excitement.

Parental Guidance Suggestions

— Teach parents that there is no really "average" baby; each is unique with its own pattern of eating, sleeping, crying, temperament, & activity.
— Encourage parents to ward off a deluge of unsolicited advice & to take their questions & concerns to one trusted, competent nurse or doctor.
— Urge parents to interview & train at least 2 or 3 mature, reliable baby sitters, or to use licensed child care persons. Try to have sitter spend time with baby while mother is there. Have mother fully explain & demonstrate details of baby's routine, as well as special likes & dislikes. Encourage mother to employ, when possible, healthy persons who are nonsmokers.

— Hold baby for feedings, looking down at baby (not at book or TV) because baby is perplexed by profile or side view of face.

— Turn situations of feeding, dressing, bathing, & diapering into pleasurable "play" situations.
Encourage water play during bath time. Pick up baby's legs & move them in circles while singing a song or saying a rhyme. Baby likes being nude, being stroked, massaged, & tickled *slightly*. Hold baby & dance to music while humming or singing along.

Common Behaviors
Three Months

— **Movement:** moves arms & legs vigorously; begins purposeful movements; when on stomach, raises head & chest, supported by forearms; holds hands in front & stares at them, wiggling fingers; reaches for objects, bringing hands together in front; puts hands & objects in mouth. Coordinates looking/grasping/sucking movements.

— **Play:** similar to that of a 2 month old.

— **Crying:** less.

— **Smiling:** more spontaneously.

— **Vocalization:** babbles and coos in response to sounds. Begins to localize sounds, voluntarily turning toward them; distinguishes speech sounds from other sounds & responds.

— **Sleep:** 16–20 hours/day; may sleep 10 hours at night, although may awaken & fret; will fall back to sleep if left undisturbed.

Parental Guidance Suggestions

— Call US Consumer Product Safety Commission (Washington, DC 20207), (800)492-2937, for booklets of information on safety standards for cribs, toys, auto seats, & accessories for children.

— Keep diaper pins & other small, loose objects out of baby's reach.

— Move baby from bassinette to a full-sized crib & from mother's bedroom to another room if this has not yet been done. Establish satisfactory sleep patterns by using crib only for sleep, by avoiding stimulation just before bedtime, by setting a consistent habit of pre-sleeping activities, & by putting baby in preferred sleep position. Rock, cuddle, hum, or play soft music, but avoid putting baby to bed with a propped bottle, as this will foster dental caries & promote association of feeding with bedtime.

— Babies who sleep on their stomach "nest" down, appearing to burrow into mattress; therefore be sure mattress is firm with no loose plastic sheets or pillows to cause smothering.

Common Behaviors
Four Months

— **Movement:** head is held steady & erect for a short time; lifts head & shoulders off surface at 90° angle when prone; supports body with hands. Rolls from back to abdomen & from stomach to side, gradually able to go from stomach to back. Begins "swimming" motions preliminary to creeping & crawling. Picks up objects with whole hand, or may take small objects between index & second fingers.

— **Play:** likes brightly colored rings, large plastic or wooden beads, spoons, keys, noisemakers. Shows preference for certain toys or blankets.

— **Smell:** distinguishes between & shows interest in different smells.

— **Vision:** eyes can focus at different lengths & follow different objects for 180°. Stares at place from which an object drops; discriminates between familiar & strange faces, responding with more pleasure to familiar, smiling faces than strangers.

— **Appearance:** birth hair is being gradually replaced by permanent hair. Eye color is changing to permanent color (although some babies will retain blue eyes up to 2 years before changing color).

— **Socialization:** likes attention, having people around to handle, play, & talk to him; becomes fussy, demanding, or bored if ignored. Enjoys sitting up & being part of a busy environment. Listens, recognizes voices, turns head toward sounds; is quiet & attentive to music.

Parental Guidance Suggestions

— Never leave infant alone on bed, table, or sofa; always use playpen, crib with rails up, or an infant seat that is securely anchored.

— Take baby for second DPT immunization.

— Hold toys within child's vision so s/he can reach for them, but don't put on string that can strangle a neck or wrist. Toys should be safe for chewing but not able to be swallowed.

— Provide opportunities for baby to smell different foods, fragrances, etc.

Common Behaviors

— **Vocalization:** expresses moods of enjoyment or protest; makes sounds, laughs, gurgles, or shrieks; laughs in response to light tickling.

— **Sleep:** sleeps through nights for up to 10 or 11 hours (although some babies will continue to wake at night & demand a feeding for as long as a year).

— **Feeding:** needs approximately 110 calories/kg/day; learning to eat from a spoon is possible now.

Parental Guidance Suggestions

— Breastfeeding continues through the 1st year; formula feeding should also continue, although evaporated milk may replace commercial formulas. Avoid over-feeding or excessive calories. Although some pediatricians still recommend low fat milk, the National Nutrition Council says that whole milk is necessary to supply essential fatty acids. Since many infants cannot properly utilize whole milk without difficulty, evaporated (heat treated) or commercial formulas should be used through the 1st year.

— 4 months is now recommended for beginning to introduce solid foods, one at a time, each week, watching carefully for allergies or intolerances (rashes, vomiting, diarrhea). Begin with single-grain enriched cereals: rice, barley, oatmeal (hold off on wheat, corn cereals, or mixed grain cereals for several weeks.)

— Don't force feed, keep mealtime pleasant, happy; let baby play with spoon, get used to smell & taste of new food as well as feel in mouth.

— Give vitamin supplements as directed; fluoride supplements may be needed if water supply for homemade formula is not fluoridated. Breastfed infants need fluoride supplements.

Common Behaviors

Five and Six Months
— **Movement:** sits momentarily without support in forward-leaning position, gradually extending time able to sit.
Hitches (moves backward in a sitting position).
Begins creeping (moves along with abdomen on floor).
Gradually able to roll completely over, from stomach to back to stomach.
Touches knees, brings feet to mouth; can be pulled up to standing position easily.
Tonic neck reflex disappears.

— **Play:** enjoys jolly-jumper, bouncer, or walker to exercise limbs & to observe environment.
Likes to look at self in mirror.
Enjoys bath & noisy water toys.
Likes large soft balls & musical balls.
Has longer attention span; can roll, play with toys for an hour or so.
Shows interest in books, pictures, paper; likes being read nursery rhymes.
Loves social games (peek-a-boo, pat-a-cake, piggy-went-to-market, etc.).

— **Socialization:** distressed around strangers

Parental Guidance Suggestions
— Sucking need is still strong, so supplement feedings with bottle of water or formula; if using pacifier, NEVER put it on a string around baby's neck or attached to its gown.

— Likes to sit in high chair to watch family activity. Enjoys outings in carriage or stroller; be sure to strap in safely; use harness in carriage or food shopping cart.
— Keep floor clear of small & dangerous objects; keep cords out of reach; cap all unused electrical outlets.
— Close off open stairwells; block off unsafe step-downs.

Common Behaviors
— **Vocalization:** utters syllables such as "ma," "ba," "da," adding new ones each week; crows, squeals, grunts, purrs, clicks, coughs, babbles.
— **Feeding:** begins to finger-feed, hold bottle & spoon.

Parental Guidance Suggestions

— Limit formula amounts to approximately 20–24 oz daily, while increasing solids to meet development & weight needs.
— Add vegetables & fruits, 1 new one each week, checking for food allergies & intolerances (rashes, vomiting, diarrhea).
— Neither approve nor scold the spitting back or blowing of food; be persistent & encouraging, patiently spooning food off face & chin or bib back into mouth.
— Realize that amounts & portions of foods vary depending on the baby's size, activity, health status, & appetite, as well as the number of other foods taken & amount of formula given. Offer bottle after eating solids.
— Allow baby to be part of family at mealtime; provide with finger-food.

Seven to Twelve Months

Physical Development
— **Weight:** gain after 6 months slows to approximately 4–5 oz per week.
— **Height:** approximately 26–28" at 6 months; grows ½"/month.

Nursing Implications and Parental Guidance Suggestions
— Evaluate child's growth status in terms of self; comparisons with charts or siblings may be inappropriate.
— Arrange for 6 months check-up and immunizations (5 months: 2nd TOPV; 6 months: 3rd DPT & TOPV).
— Because of baby's rejection of strangers at this time, try to do as much of the exam as possible while baby is sitting in mother's lap. Proceed with the less distressing tasks first, giving baby something to interest & distract him. Remember to smile & talk to baby while conducting examination.

Physical Development
— **Teeth:** begin to erupt around 6 months; 2 central lower incisors first, then 2 central upper incisors, then upper & lower lateral incisors.

Common Behaviors
Seven to Nine Months
— **Movement:** toe sucking common; preference for right or left handedness occurs. Sits alone well by 9 months. Raises self to sitting position. Tries various ways to move body; some may crawl (on all 4 limbs with abdomen up off floor). May start pulling self to a stand, learning later how to return to floor. Bounces & bears some weight in standing position.

Nursing Implications and Parental Guidance Suggestions
— Prior to eruption, baby's gums are swollen & tender; baby is irritable & restless, may have slight fever or change in bowel habits. Mother can rub gums with finger, a cold spoon, or chilled teething rings. Sometimes the dentist will prescribe a medication to numb the gums. Symptoms subside when teeth erupt. Parents should know that high fever, diarrhea, or upper respiratory symptoms are not teething symptoms; these illnesses should be reported promptly to doctor.
— Show mother how to clean newly erupted teeth of placque by using a clean washcloth. "Baby" teeth or primary teeth are important for chewing, for appearance, for proper development of jaws & mouth, & for reserving space for permanent teeth. Placque & decay need prompt care to control. "Nursing bottle" decay occurs when naptime or bedtime bottles of sweetened liquids are given; the decay process begins during the sleeping hours.

Parental Guidance Suggestions

— Hand things to baby directly in front of eyes & chest; don't try to change way baby tries to grasp them.
— Keep wastebaskets hidden & out of reach; avoid pinching baby's fingers when closing doors, cupboards, drawers.
— Strap baby safely into strollers, carriages, grocery carts, high chairs. Close off stairs or teach baby how to crawl down them, feet & legs first.

Common Behaviors

— **Play:** likes large plastic & wooden blocks, nesting boxes or cups, stacking rings, water toys, paper to crumple, plastic keys, measuring cups & bowls.

— **Socialization:** wriggles & giggles in anticipation of play; learns meaning of "no" by voice tone; pats mirror image; resists doing what s/he doesn't want to do.
Wants to play in presence of family; perform for audience. Shows open & fond affection for family members; exhibits comfort around children; fear of strangers reaches peak & starts to lessen. Thinks that anything not within range of vision is gone, but is beginning to understand disappearance concept.
Imitates adult movements such as clapping, swaying, making sounds & noises.

— **Vocalization:** loves to imitate; coughs, clicks, buzzes; says syllables like "ma," "da," "ga."

— **Sleep:** 14–16 hours/24, including 1–2 daytime naps.

— **Feeding:** eats 3 meals/day; holds spoon, drinks from a cup, enjoys finger foods, tastes everything.

Parental Guidance Suggestions

— Use jolly jumper, walker, & play pen to practice standing & improve muscle tone. Play "hide-a-toy" with baby. Continue social games; give toy telephone; play music of many kinds, provide simple rhythm instruments (drum, bells, xylophone); read rhymes, poems, sing-song stories with repetitive sounds (Dr. Seuss-type) and ABC rhyme books with pictures.

— Because of stranger anxiety, cost of sitters, & baby's comfort around children, it is tempting & convenient to involve older siblings in a large amount of baby care while mother is otherwise busy; safety of baby & maturity of older child must be prime considerations, as well as possibility of sibling rivalry & the need of older child to have usual routines of after-school activities.

— Allow longer time for feeding so child can practice new skills. Show excitement at baby's achievements. May or may not show readiness for weaning; still has strong sucking needs & the emotional need to be held even though willing to hold own bottle. Gradually decrease amount & frequency of milk (formula) feedings, while increasing foods of various kinds & textures; include meat, soft pieces of fruit, cheese, toast.

Common Behaviors

Ten to Twelve Months
— **Movement:** crawls & creeps well; climbs up & down from furniture; climbs up stairs, but needs to be taught how to crawl down backwards.
Pulls self to feet; by 12 months, can stand alone for a few minutes & pivot body 90°.
"Cruises" or sidesteps along furniture (average 11 months).
Begins walking (average 12 months).
Stoops, squats, bends, leans, reaches, opens drawers, lifts lids.
Begins to help dressing self.
Can pick up objects now & can voluntarily release them. Can hold 2 or more objects in hand; can "store" object in mouth or under arm while grabbing another one.
Likes to handle, shake, bang, roll, fill, empty, push, spin, drop, & otherwise manipulate all objects.

Parental Guidance Suggestions
Avoid foods that can cause choking (raw carrots, nuts, popcorn). Start good nutritional habits by avoiding too many sweet cookies & salty crackers. Do not introduce candy or ice cream.

— Allow freedom to creep & walk in safe, baby-proof areas.
— For babies who can climb out of crib, use a net or put crib side down, placing crib next to a bed to cushion descent. Baby-proof bedroom & be sure baby cannot open door. Close off stairways or teach baby how to crawl down backwards, safely.
— Use only toy hampers without lids to prevent pinched fingers.
— Assure parents of a "quiet" baby (or one that is "late" developing motor skills) that when baby is ready, learning & practice time is often shorter than for those babies who started to crawl, climb, or walk earlier; some babies show interest in movement, others in vocalization, still others in passive study & observation.
— Whether babies should learn to walk in bare feet or soft or hard-soled shoes is controversial. Consult pediatrician & consider own needs & environment. When purchasing shoes, buy them only ½" longer & ¼" wider than baby's foot to allow natural spread & growth. Too large shoes are clumsy, cause blisters, & force unnatural foot position to develop. Too small shoes also cause problems, so check size & fit at least monthly.

Common Behaviors

Parental Guidance Suggestions

Minor toeing-in is normal for the new walker & can correct itself when baby's balance is better.

Some doctors recommend temporarily putting shoes on "wrong" feet for a month or 2.

— Teach baby meaning of "hot" & "don't touch." Set firm, consistent limits.

Try to be patient & persevering. Join a parent support group for mutual aid & help.

— Show love openly; touch, hold, rock, be active with child.

— Supervise older children "sitting" with or playing with baby, so they don't frighten or inadvertently hurt baby; help older children express frustrations at baby's behavior in socially acceptable & safe ways. Do things as a family, showing love & respect for older child's needs.

— **Play:** likes rocking horse & riding toys. Likes to play chase. Prefers push toys to pull toys. Likes to rock, sway, keep time & "dance" with someone to music.

— Provide new & different toys that stimulate curiosity like milk cartons, fabric or cardboard boxes, containers to fill and spill, pots, etc.

— Don't pretend to be something fearful or jump out at baby with loud noises.

— Play music in baby's bedroom or playroom.

— **Socialization:** may begin temper tantrums. Seeks approval but is not always cooperative. Shaking head "no" is easier than nodding "yes." Shows moods.

— Walk away from baby having a temper tantrum, or place in own room with door closed. Reward verbally for cooperative behavior.

— **Verbalization:** responds to own name. Can identify (by pointing to) objects such as sky, airplane, familiar animals, & people. May be able to say 3 or 4 words ("ma-ma," "no," "hi," "hot").

— Be alert to detect early hearing losses. See a pediatric audiologist if baby does not respond to own name, cannot imitate simple sounds, or cannot point to familiar objects.

Common Behaviors

— **Sleeping:** some active babies sleep only 11–12 hours at night with 1 hour daytime nap. Some babies still wake at night to stand, to be rocked, to have a bottle.

— **Feeding:** will eat less solid food if formula or breastfeeding not correspondingly reduced; gains less weight as movement increases.

Parental Guidance Suggestions

— Don't force baby to eat more than s/he wants or force foods that baby dislikes. Allow longer mealtime if baby is feeding self. Allow baby to use fingers & don't force spoon usage at all times. Give baby a spillproof plastic cup; a plastic sheet or newspapers on floor during mealtimes will ease cleanup of spills.

Twelve to Eighteen Months

Physical Development

— **Weight:** average 20–24 lbs, triples birth weight by 12 months, gaining 2–6 lbs in next 6 months.

— **Height:** approximately 29'' growing to approximately 33'' by 18 months.

— **Size:** head and chest circumference are about equal at 12 months.

— **Pulse:** 100–140/minute. **Respirations:** 20–40/minute.

— **Reflexes:** Babinski sign disappears.

— **Anterior Fontanel:** closes (average 10–24 months).

— **Abdomen:** protrudes.

— **Teething:** continues with 10–14 primary teeth by 18 months, including lower & upper molars & cuspids. Good chewing, sucking, & swallowing movements.

Nursing Implications and Parental Guidance Suggestions

— Recommend 1 year physical check-up, with Hgb., Hct., urinalysis.

— At 15 months give measles, mumps, & rubella vaccines, & TB skin test.

— At 18 months give DPT & TOPV boosters.

— Measure vital signs at rest.

— Evaluate fontanel & cranial configurations.

— Urge dental hygiene (brushing, fluoridated drops, toothpaste).

Common Behaviors
— **Movement:** able to walk alone with a widebased gait.
  Climbs upstairs, holding onto hand or rail, 1 step at a time.
  Throws, turns pages in a book, builds a tower of 3 objects/
  blocks.
  Helps in dressing self with hat, shoes, lifting arms or legs
  appropriately.

— **Play:** likes large cars & trucks, dolls, mops, brooms, kitchen
  utensils, stuffed animals, 2–10 piece puzzles, balls, picture
  books.
  Loves to throw & retrieve objects. Delights in pushing, pulling, or riding toys; climbing up, down, & through indoor
  gym/slide combinations.
  Enjoys solitary play or watching others.

— **Socialization:** explores everything with rapid attention shifts.
  Curious; trial & error behavior; learns s/he can control some
  things around self; enjoys new skills; shows pride in
  achievements.
  Imitates & mimics household chores.
  Security is focused on one object (doll, blanket, stuffed
  animal, thumb, diaper).

Parental Guidance Suggestions
— Protect child from kitchen accidents (hot liquids, over-
  hanging handles, cords on appliances, long table cloths).
  Lock up all medicines, poisons, gasoline, fertilizers, cleaning agents. Check all houseplants, keeping them out of
  reach; discard poisonous varieties. Keep matches out of
  reach. Put safety plugs in electrical outlets. Supervise yard
  play. Never leave alone in bath water, wading, or other
  pools. Always use seat belts & approved car seats. Use safety devices on cabinet drawers & all doors.

— Know that the parents' reaction to child's failure (or accomplishments) affects the child's self-concept. Showing anxiety over minor injuries, anger at childish carelessness, or ig-
  noring accomplishments can have an unhealthful effect on
  child's self-esteem. Try to treat minor injuries, failures, with
  casual acceptance. Show pleasure at new social or physical
  skills.

Common Behaviors
— **Verbalization:** can point to parts of body when asked; can say 3–12 meaningful single words: "ma-ma," "da-da," "no," "hi," "hot," "bye-bye," "go," "baby," "wa-wa" (water), "ball," "dis" (this), "dat" (that), "cookie," "car." Begins to follow a few simple commands, e.g,, "Give it to me," "Show me the ___."
— **Elimination:** may be able to control BMs or void at will on potty chair, but usually not interested.
— **Feeding:** feeds self with spoon & drinks from cup by 18 months; appetite decreases with decreasing growth rate. Needs 100 calories/kg or approximately 1300/day (range: 900–1800 calories).

Parental Guidance Suggestions
— Set firm, safe limits.

— Delay weaning & bowel or bladder training until baby's readiness evident (shows interest & cooperation).

— If growth rate is proceeding normally as determined by pediatrician, don't force feed, coax, wheedle, bribe, threaten, or punish poor appetite or feeding. Give regular table foods in a 3-meal-a-day pattern with nutritious between-meal or bed-time snacks. Give *very small* helpings. Keep child at table only as long as interested in eating. Do not give snacks *as an alternative* to mealtime eating. Do not appease a fussy or crying baby with a cookie or sweets. Do not use food as a reward, as a comfort for small hurts, or as a substitute for love & attention.

Recommended References
Baby and Child Care, by Dr. B. Spock. New York: Pocket Books, 1977.
Becoming a Father, by S. Gresh. New York: Butterick Publishing, 1980.
Best Practical Parenting Tips—First Five Years, by V. Lansky. Wayzata, MN: Meadowbrook Press, 1980.
"Dad's Point of View," by L. Woolfe. *Baby Talk*, February 1982:24–28, 50, 51.
"A Developmental Approach to Physical Assessment," by L. Yoos. *MCN: The American Journal of Maternal Child Nursing*, May/June 1981:168–170.
"The First Year of Life." *American Baby*, Mid-February 1981:35–132.
Kids are Fragile—Travel with Care. Bothell, WA: Action for Child Transportation Safety (ACTS), Child Restraint Committee (PO Box 266, 98011).
"Normal Growth and Development: Neonate." *NCP Guide #3:22*, 2nd Ed., Nurseco, 1983.
Principles and Techniques in Pediatric Nursing, 4th Ed., by G. Leifer. Philadelphia: Saunders, 1982.
"Watching Baby's Diet: A Professional and Parental Guide," by B. Markesbery and W. Wong. *MCN: Journal of Maternal Child Nursing*, May/June 1979:177–180.

Normal Growth & Development: Toddler and Pre-Schooler

Definition: Toddlerhood is the developmental period in a child's life between one and three years. Pre-school covers from three to six years of age.

LONG TERM GOAL: The child will achieve the highest level of potential growth and development; the child will develop an autonomous personality and self-confident abilities within the family; by the time the child enters school or kindergarten, s/he will:
  1) have had an eye screening test and scored within norms, or have vision corrected;
  2) have had a hearing test and scored within norms;
  3) have passed a DDST (Denver Developmental Screening Test) for age at an acceptable level;
  4) have received all legally required immunizations (list here for your state);
  5) have a record of regular physical examinations and have all current known health problems under medical or nursing supervision;
  6) have a dental record of yearly examinations and treatment;
  7) be able to demonstrate basic oral hygiene skills and general hygiene practices (handwashing, use of tissues for nasal discharge, covering mouth for coughs and sneezes); and
  8) have passed a kindergarten readiness test at an acceptable level or be scheduled to receive special educational assistance.

General Considerations:
— **Rate of growth and development as well as task mastery** varies with each individual child. Parental and environmental influences may stimulate and nurture or retard development, but innate differences and individual readiness will strongly affect level and rate of achievement.
— **Developmental task** (Erikson's central problem) to be resolved during *toddlerhood* is *autonomy* or independence *versus shame* or doubt, and during the *pre-school* period it is *initiative versus guilt*. Successfully achieved, the youngster develops pride, high self-esteem, and good will to self and others.

— **Special fears** of toddlers and pre-schoolers are those of abandonment and separation from parents. Learning to separate from parents and to cope effectively is an important task of the young child. Success can be achieved when the child experiences positive periods of short separation and feels trust and security with those who care for him. Coping skills begin to include modes of self-expression and elementary self-reliance. Familiar surroundings and mother's presence are no longer always necessary for the child to feel secure.

— **Cognitive abilities** develop rapidly in the pre-school years and the child learns many things. The toddler has a concept of time limited to the present experience, focuses on only one aspect of objects, problem solves through trial and error, imitates language heard, and perceives through senses. Piaget calls this the "sensorimotor" stage of cognitive development. The pre-schooler's thinking is termed "preoperational," is literal, concrete, and absolute (good/bad, right/wrong, hurt/doesn't hurt, etc.). S/he views the world and people's actions in terms of own self and consequences to self, refusing others' viewpoints. The pre-schooler asks "why" and "how" frequently, extends concept of time to include past as well as present, and has a longer memory span than toddlers.

— **Imagination** is heightened in the pre-schooler; fantasy and reality are often interchangeable. Imaginary companions people this fantasy world, are often blamed for the youngster's own misbehavior, and serve as coping mechanisms for controlling situations, especially stressful ones.

— **Play** in the toddler period is active, informal, spontaneous, and often centered around motor activity. Characteristically, toddler play is singular and referred to as *parallel play* (when two children play alongside but not with each other). When the child learns to give in order to receive, s/he makes the transition into the pre-school type of play known as *cooperative or associative play*.

— **Ritualism** is a common behavioral pattern of these two periods; activities of daily living are best scheduled and performed precisely and regularly in order to provide security and stability for the child in a rapidly changing period of growth and development.

— **Negativism** and the consistent use of the word "NO" for everything is characteristic of this period. It is the toddlers' way of controlling people and events, acting on their own terms, doing things by themselves (*"Me* do it myself!"); the negative response becomes quite an automatic one.

— **Temper tantrums** are the young child's way of expressing frustration and releasing anger at people, things, and self in an effort to gain control. An angry, kicking toddler in the midst of a tantrum cannot be effectively dealt with by threats or reasoning for s/he is oblivious to reality. Walk away from a child having a tantrum; do not be a sympathetic or angry bystander; reward verbally for cooperative, socially acceptable behavior.

— The **common parameters** of physical development and behaviors for the toddler and pre-school child are outlined below, together with corresponding nursing implications and teaching or guidance suggestions.

Eighteen Months to Three Years

Physical Development	Nursing Implications and Parental Guidance Suggestions

Physical Development
— **Weight:** average 28–30 lbs (13 kg)
— **Height:** average 33–37"

Nursing Implications and Parental Guidance Suggestions
— Caution parents that appetite & weight gain level off during this period; thus child can eat less & still maintain activity levels. 1980 revised RDA recommended energy requirements for the toddler are 900–1800 calories/day (average 1300). Provide appropriate counselling &/or evaluation for children above 95th percentile or below 5th percentile for height or weight. Any child whose pattern has changed markedly (e.g., from 50th to 10th percentile or vice versa) also should be further evaluated.
Check all measurements & ascertain that they were accurately taken. Norms are based on children being weighed with no clothing except light undergarments.

— **Pulse:** 90–120/minute. **Respirations:** 20–35/minute.

— Count for 1 full minute.

— **Teeth:** 16 at 2 years, acquiring a full set of 20 primary teeth by 3 years.

— Establish nutritious, non-cariogenic dietary & snacking habits for proper tooth formation & bone development. Offer pretzels, fruits, fruit juice, & raw vegetables. Avoid carrot sticks, popcorn, & nuts because of possible choking. Keep candy, cookies, raisins, pastries, sweetened soft drinks & gum to a minimum.
— Take child for 1st dental visit by age 2 or before all 20 primary teeth have erupted. Take to dentist immediately for any cavities noticed or injuries to teeth. Make first dental visit a pleasant, friendly one, preparing child with a positive, matter-of-fact explanation. Read child a book about visiting the dentist. Remember that parental attitudes & examples can mold a child's feelings about dental care for many years.

Physical Development

— **Vision:** visual acuity is approximately 20/70 in the 2 year old.

— **Body proportions:** changing, with abdomen protruding, arms and legs lengthening rapidly, and trunk and head growing slowly.

Common Behaviors
Two Year Old
— **Movement:** gait is steady; walks, runs, jumps with both feet. Climbs stairs 1 at a time with both feet on each step, holding rail. Can open doors & turn knobs. Can kick a ball without falling, even when running.

Nursing Implications and Parental Guidance Suggestions

Cleaning (brushing & flossing) teeth properly is a skill mastered over time; it requires careful teaching, demonstration, & supervision for several years or longer depending on the individual child. Topical fluoridation treatments may be applied for additional decay protection. Continue fluoride supplements for children who do not live in a community with fluoridated water supply.

— Since nearly 1 out of 5 children have visual disorders that often go undetected even by observant parents, a complete eye exam by a specialist is recommended for every child between 1 & 3 years of age.

— A free brochure on children's vision is available from The Children's Eyesight Society, 7420 Westlake Terrace, Suite 1509, Bethesda, MD 20034.

— Falls & stumbling may increase during this period due to changing body proportions & rapidly increasing motor skills. In addition, toddlers assert autonomy & overestimate physical capabilities. Supervision & precautions are necessary to minimize accidents (install stairway rails, sturdy high fences; remove loose throw rugs, tables with sharp edges, glass objects that can topple over).

Parental Guidance Suggestions

— Carefully supervise all outdoor & indoor play.
— Teach child street & traffic safety.
— Use fire retardant night clothes.
— Lock up all dangerous products.

Common Behaviors

By 2½ can ride a "kiddy" car & tricycle. Can throw objects overhead, string large beads, & begin to use scissors. Can scribble & copy vertical & straight lines.

Assists with dressing & undressing self.

Washes & dries hands. Uses toothbrush, but not skillfully.

— **Play:** has short attention span; needs combination of motor activities with quiet play. Enjoys stories, music, TV, sandbox with toys, Play-doh, clay, mud, & finger-paints. Likes construction toys, cars, trucks, pull toys, wagons, doll buggies, and riding toys like fire engines, tricycles, kiddy cars. Enjoys climbing & swinging playground apparatus, puzzles with large pieces, drawing paper, musical & rhythm instruments, dolls, stuffed animals, & toy household items for imitative play (brooms, lawnmowers, etc.). Parallel play predominates.

— **Socialization:** is egocentric, the center of own world, viewing all in relationship to self. Treats other children almost as if they were objects.

May bite in anger or frustration or just to use teeth.

Other frequently observed behaviors include self-stimulation (rocking, masturbation), thumbsucking, ritualism, & negativism.

Parental Guidance Suggestions

— Lock doors or put plastic holders over doorknobs to prevent toddler usage.

— Use car seats every time.

— Post a poison chart with poison control center phone number.

— Supervise water play constantly.

— Begin swim lessons if pool is present & accessible, even occasionally.

— Make sure riding toys are in good working order.

— Child has a need for peer companionship, even if unable to share. Do not expect child to do more than s/he is able to do.

— Biting back, slapping, shouting, or putting something unpleasant in mouth (like soap or hot sauce) usually do not work. Verbal disapproval, removal of child from stressor, or addressing cause (e.g., sibling rivalry) will at least have some positive effect.

— Accept the normalcy of behavior for this stage. Remain consistent in discipline; provide periods of special quiet time alone with child, reading stories, playing music, cuddling, & providing individual attention.

— Give choices when possible. Do not offer choices where none are present.

Common Behaviors

— **Verbalization:** has speaking vocabulary of 20 + words & understands hundreds more. Begins using phrases of 2–4 words (e.g., "go bye-bye," "more cookie," "where daddy," "me do it"). Most popular words: "no,", "me," "my," "mine."

— **Elimination:** may gradually become toilet-trained at least during daytime.

Parental Guidance Suggestions

— Introduce toilet training if child shows signs of readiness (ability to stand & walk well, hold urine for 2 hours at a time, regular schedule of bowel movements, willingness to please caregiver, ability to indicate need to eliminate).

— Do not start toilet training during stressful periods (birth of a sibling, weaning, moving, family separations, illness).

— Teaching should be positive, pleasant, non-punitive, non-pressured, & geared to the particular child.

— Expect accidents when child is tired, excited, preoccupied, busy with play, or otherwise in a stressful situation. React casually & noncommittally.

— Keep potty chair accessible or a step stool near a standard toilet fitted with a smaller seat adaptation.

— Be consistent in reinforcements (rewards); use praise, not sweets. Use correct terminology for body parts. Begin foundation for health sex education; refrain from negative responses for normal curiosity. Child may want to see elimination products or not want them flushed away immediately; postpone it temporarily.

— Use loose fitting, easily removed outer clothing & training pants that child can manage without help.

— **Sleeping:** 10–14 hours/day, including an afternoon nap.

— **Feeding:** requires approximately 1300 calories/day. Feeds self without spilling.

— Keep portions small; choose foods from basic 4 food groups.

Three Years to Six Years

Physical Development

— **Weight:** approximately 44 lbs (*at least* 5 times birth weight by 5 years)

— **Height:** approximately 44" (about double birth length and ⅔ adult height)

— **Pulse:** 80–120/minute. **Respirations:** 20–30/minute.

— **BP:** 85–90/60 mm Hg.

— **Teeth:** begins to lose primary teeth at approximately 5–7 years.

— **Immunizations:** boosters needed for DPT & TOPV.

— **Vision:** visual acuity is approximately 20/40 in 3 year old, 20/30 in 4 year old, & normal 20/20 by age 6. Depth perception is developing & color vision fully established.

— **Body proportions:** loses much of baby fat & protruding abdomen; waist not discernible; legs continue to grow rapidly equaling approximately 44% of total length.

Common Behaviors
Three Year Old

— **Movement:** climbs stairs, alternating feet, but still holding rail. Tries to draw a picture, a mass of lines & circles. Can hit

Nursing Implications and Parental Guidance Suggestions

— Same as above, for toddler.

— Height & weight are about even at age 5.

— Count for 1 full minute.

— Use child-size blood pressure cuff. Let child handle equipment & listen to own heart beat. Blood pressure determinations are a regular part of the physical exam beginning at age 3; plot on a normative pediatric graph; successive readings above the 95th percentile require further follow-up evaluation.

— Evaluate physical conditioning, immunization, vision, hearing, & kindergarten readiness skills before starting school; provide appropriate corrections & assistance.

Parental Guidance Suggestions

— Continue supervision & safety precautions, even though child shows signs of using more caution & responsibility.

Common Behaviors

a pegboard with a hammer with more accuracy than before. Dresses self with help on grippers, zippers, buttons, & shoe tying.

Can help with minor tasks such as drying dishes, emptying waste baskets, getting or putting away items such as cleaning utensils or groceries.

— **Play:** uses blackboard & chalk, Dressy Bessy-type doll, housekeeping toys, windup musical toys, child's typewriter, record player, tape player, mechanical games, increasing numbers & varieties of books, puzzles, trucks, building toys.

— **Socialization:** can tolerate short periods of separation, especially if child is in a happy, play-type situation with competent adults.

— **Verbalization:** has mastered most vowels, half the consonents; speaks in short sentences that are becoming more complex. Has a rapidly expanding speaking vocabulary of 300 + words; understands many more words than this. Frequently repeats words & syllables as a means of learning them. 90% of 3 year olds should be readily understood by others.

Questions everything with "what?" "when?" "why?" & "how?" Understands simple explanations of cause & effect.

Parental Guidance Suggestions

— Teach child what to do if lost while shopping or in new situation. Provide ID bracelet. Teach child name, age, & phone number.

— Give small errands or jobs to do around house. Watch & wait before offering help or suggestions.

— Expand child's world with same age group play experiences (babysitting co-ops or playgroups, nursery school or Sunday school situations, trips to zoo, playgrounds, story hours, etc.)

— Encourage development of cooperative, sharing, or associative play skills.

— Encourage child to express feelings verbally & accept feelings, while redirecting unacceptable behavior to more acceptable behavior.

— Parents can help develop child's language skills by talking aloud about what one is doing, thinking, & feeling; also by "parallel" talk describing what someone else may be doing, thinking, feeling while it happens.

— Patiently provide simple but honest explanations upon request. Show & describe how things work & why something is dangerous or unwise to handle.

Common Behaviors
— **Elimination:** goes to bathroom with minimal help.

— **Sleeping & Feeding:** similar to 2 year old.

Four Year Old
— **Movement:** walks with a freeswinging, adult-like stride; walks backwards; can walk upstairs without grasping rail. Can stand on 1 foot for 5 seconds. Runs well. Hops 2 or more times. Throws ball overhead with control & increasing accuracy to someone. Uses scissors to cut out pictures, following outline with increasing accuracy. Can draw a picture of a person with head, eyes, & 2 other parts.

— **Play:** is cooperative; dramatic, imitative play predominates. May have an imaginary companion. Likes jumpropes; play tools; paste & various scraps (cloth, leaves, paper) to arrange in collage; easels with paints; tires & very large boxes to climb around in; gym sets.

— **Socialization:** brags, shows off, looks for praise, criticizes others, tattles. Developing a conscience that influences behavior.
Develops romantic fantasies about parents of opposite sex. Common age for nightmares, castration fears, fears of scary objects & animals.

Parental Guidance Suggestions
— Remind child to go before going outside or when playing busily.

— Check play areas to remove unsafe hazards. Clear trash heaps; cover holes, ditches, tunnels; lock empty refrigerators or remove doors; properly discard faulty appliances, paint cans, plastic bags, aerosol cans.

— Provide dressup clothing for imitative play (cowboy hats, guns, holster, purses, jewelry, adult clothes).
— Take to children's plays, musical performances, puppet shows.
— Enroll in dance classes, swim lessons, exercise classes, & other learning opportunities.

— Invite friends over for parties, play activities, group games.

— Because of nightmares at this age, child may want to sleep with parent. Start child in own bed, perhaps with light on & relaxing music. Temporary cuddling in parents' bed for nightmares can be condoned, but when child falls asleep, return to own bed. Patience & persistence, along with growing out of this stage will return the child to a regular, secure sleeping routine.

Common Behaviors

— **Verbalization:** has a speaking vocabulary of 1000 + words, expanding approximately 600 words/year depending on stimulation by adults & older siblings.
Talks incessantly; knows own name, age, phone number, & some know address.
Scatology appears now (the use of socially unacceptable words for their shock effect).
Knows primary colors & some numbers & alphabet letters.

— **Sleeping:** 11–12 hours/day, napping only occasionally when very tired or ill.

— **Feeding:** requires approximately 1700 calories/day (range: 1300–2300 calories/day) for 4–6 year olds.

Five Years Old

— **Movement:** can run & play games at same time; hops & skips well; some may attempt to ride a 2-wheel bicycle without training wheels, but this skill comes gradually to those closer to 6 years. May begin rollerskating, iceskating, & skiing. May be able to swim standard swim strokes a distance of 25 yards.
Begins to use fork & knife.
May be able to print first name, sometimes a short last name.
Some may be able to tie shoelaces, but many are unable to do this until 6–8 years.
Draws a recognizable person with body, head, arms, legs, & four other parts.

Parental Guidance Suggestions

— Reinforce new knowledge with toys, games, books about numbers, colors, & letters.

— Teach safe use of toys & riding or moving equipment (bikes, skates, skateboards, etc.).
— Teach safe street crossing, obeying traffic lights & cross-walk lines.
— Teach child how to phone for help (fire, police, paramedics, emergency 911).
— Teach child to recite name, age, phone number, & address.

Common Behaviors

Can count to 20 & may recognize coinage of a penny, nickel, dime.

Can wash self without wetting clothes.

Can brush teeth correctly with reminders & some supervision.

— **Play:** can use rollerskates, iceskates, sleds, scooters, skateboards, riding toys. Likes building sets, toy soldiers, plastic people, toy animals, doll houses.

— **Socialization:** takes some responsibility for actions, following directions & rules. Increased respect for truth. Growth of modesty & wish for privacy. Able to sit quietly for 10–15 minutes to hear a story or lesson. Interested in meaning of family relationships (aunts, uncles, cousins, grandparents).

— **Verbalization:** has a vocabulary of 2000 + words. Can explain to others how & why of games or activities. Begins sentences with "I" instead of "me;" "he" instead of "him."

Parental Guidance Suggestions

— Add more books, games, puzzles, involving increasing manipulative & cognitive skills.

— Teach child never to talk with strangers or to enter strange cars, either alone or with other playmates.

— Keep behavior rules simple, enforce consistently; avoid prolonged arguments.

— Keep in close touch with kindergarten teacher to learn more about child's progress, abilities, needs, & to get suggestions for helping & guiding child. Help to build child's self-confidence by praising new skills, positive attitudes, & acceptable behavior.

— Although child may mispronounce some sounds & make some grammatical errors, most of the time his language should closely match that of the family & neighborhood. For suspected problems, get further evaluation from MD.

Recommended References

"Caring For Your Children's Teeth." *Consumer's Guide to Dental Health 1982*, special issue of *The Journal of the American Dental Association*:19C–26C.

Food Before Six. Rosemont, IL: National Dairy Council (6300 N. River Road, 60018).

"The Independent Toddler," by S. Scott. *American Baby*, May 1981:43–50.

Learning to Talk—Speech, Hearing, and Language Problems in the Pre-School Child. Bethesda, MD: Office of Scientific and Health Reports, National Institutes of Health, 1977.

When Your Child is Contrary, Why Children Don't Eat and What to do About It, Your Child's Appetite, Your Child's Fears, Developing Toilet Habits, Your Child and Sleep Problems, and other pamphlets for parents. Columbus, OH: Ross Laboratories Creative Services and Information Department (625 N. Cleveland Avenue, 43216).

Normal Growth & Development: School-Age Child

Definition: The school years are the developmental period in an child's life between six and eleven years of age.

LONG TERM GOAL: The child will develop his maximum potential within the framework of his family, peers, and the school environment; the child will develop a beginning understanding of himself, his relationship to others, and the world around him.

General Considerations:

— **Developmental task** (Erikson's central problem) to be resolved during this period is *industry* versus *inferiority*. The child moves out into many different social groups and, while the family remains the chief socializing agent, s/he learns new and important skills and attitudes from peers: (1) the art of compromise, cooperation, and persuasion; (2) fair play through competition; (3) increased autonomy from the home; (4) reinforcement of appropriate sex-role behaviors; and (5) an ongoing development of self-concept.

— **Cognitive development:** time is now well understood and the child can plan ahead. There is a mature concept of causality. Formal logical thinking is present. The child expands his knowledge rapidly through formal and informal educational means. The child begins to combine others' viewpoints with his own. S/he is capable of prolonged interest and attention span. The memory is good for concrete sequences of numbers and letters and for two meaningful and related ideas.

— **Egocentrism** continues during this period. A form of "cognitive conceit" assures the child that s/he is always right; it is also shocking when they realize that parents are fallible and that they (or teachers) are *not always* right. This conceit can occasionally create in a child an ambivalence about growing up to be an imperfect adult; this, and other worries, results sometimes in compulsive nervous habits like nail biting, hair twisting, other mannerisms, or nightmares. Special fears of this period are those of bodily injury, concern about death, fear of parental loss, and fear of embarrassment from criticism or ridicule.

— **Play** is centered around groups of same sex after six or seven years of age; "gang" activities predominate in both school and recreational interests (clubs, teams, scouts, parties, enrichment classes, neighborhood play groups). Peer group influence becomes important and peer criticism begins for deviation from sex roles, intellectual or physical skill differences, socio-cultural differences, and noncomformity in language, dress, social behaviors. Quarrels are frequent but usually short-lived. The school age child has now learned to share and take turns and can participate in organized games requiring coordinated efforts.

— The **common parameters** of physical development and behaviors for the school-age child are outlined below, together with corresponding nursing implications and teaching or guidance suggestions.

Six to Eleven Years

Physical Development

— **Weight:** 45 lbs (20 kg) at 6 years, child gains 5–7lbs/year on average; 62 lbs (28 kg) at 7–10 years.

— **Height:** 46"(117 cm) at 6 years; growth occurs in spurts; overall height averages approximately 3" (cm)/year, 52"(132 cm) at 7–10 years.

— **Pulse:** 80–100/minute at 6 years; approximates adult norm at 10–11 years. **Respirations:** 18–20/minute at 6 years; approximates adult norms at 10–11 years.

— **BP:** 95–108/60–68; approximates adult norms at 10–11 years.

— **Vision:** 20/20 by 7 years.

— **Feeding:** caloric requirements for 7–10 year old range from 1650–3300/day (average 2400 calories).

— **Teeth:** first permanent molars come in at 6–7 years; primary teeth are lost in order of eruption; has 10–11 permanent teeth by 10–11 years of age.

— **Sex Characteristics:** early development may begin in girls as soon as 8 years, & in boys as soon as 10 years.

Nursing Implications and Parental Guidance Suggestions

— Refer to growth charts as guidelines, but do not use as rigid criteria.

— Urge annual well-child check-ups.

— Verify immunization status complies with state requirements.

— Promote vision testing every 2 years.

— Encourage children to sit no closer to TV than 4'.

— Assess nutritional status & further evaluate children in the upper or lower percentiles of weight. Have parent keep food diary for 1 week (with child's help). Reinforce basic nutrition ideas & stress healthful eating habits.

— Remind parents to schedule twice-yearly dental check-ups & to continue supervision of correct brushing & flossing techniques.

— Early developers are often subject to ridicule & embarrassment. Children need education & counseling to understand & accept the changes in their bodies. Adolescent growth spurt often begins by 10–11 years but may not occur until nearly 14. See Recommended References for helping parents increase their effectiveness in providing sex education for their children.

Common Behaviors
Six Year Old
— **Movement:** large muscle ability exceeds fine motor coordination. Girls are ahead of boys in fine motor skills, physical development, & achievement. High energy levels; very active, impulsive, & constantly in motion. Balance & rhythm are good. Can hop, skip, run, jump, gallop, & climb. Can kick, throw, & catch a ball well. Can ride a 2-wheel bicycle without training wheels. Able to draw a recognizable human figure, house, flowers.
Dresses self with almost no help; can master buttons, grippers, zippers, & shoelaces.

— **Play:** plays well alone, but enjoys groups of both sexes in small groups. Likes simple games with basic rules. Likes to make things (starts many, but finishes few). Likes imaginary, dramatic play with real costumes, running games of tag, hide-and-seek, rollerskating, kickball, soccer, jumprope games, hopscotch, iceskating, skiing, & skateboarding.
Plays house; builds with plastic blocks. Still plays with dolls, airplanes, cars, & trucks. Enjoys electronic & musical games, puzzles, & books with words as well as pictures. Likes to draw, color, paint, paste, & cut.

— **Socialization:** boisterous, verbally aggressive, assertive, bossy, opinionated, outgoing, active, argumentative, sometimes whiny, & know-it-all.
Expresses sense of humor in riddles, practical jokes, & nonsense.

Parental Guidance Suggestions

— Teach & reinforce traffic safety, provide adult supervision of play.
— Teach child to avoid strangers, never get in an unknown car, never take candy, food, or pills from strangers.
— Provide for a balance of rest & activity.
— Teach cold prevention (separate drinking cups) & good health practices, including reinforcement of dangers of drug abuse & taking medicines or pills not prescribed by a physician.

— Give some responsibility for household duties within ability & maturity level.

— Assure parents that aggressiveness is normal for age; suggest sidestepping power struggles; offer choices when possible.
— Frequently reassure the child of his competence, basic worth & lovability.

Common Behaviors
Moods & feelings (fear, joy, affection, anger, shyness, jealousy, sadness) expressed in extremes.
Can use a telephone.
Has a strong need for teacher approval, affection, & acceptance.
Very aware of teacher's social attitudes & values as communicated by behavior.
Learns concepts of coinage, right & left, morning & afternoon, days of week, months of year, beginning reading & printing.
Peer group influence also becoming important.

— **Verbalization:** has a vocabulary of 2–3000 words. Communicates to share thoughts & ideas with others. Understanding of language greater than ability to use it. Can verbalize similarities.

— **Eating:** needs approximately 2000 calories/day. Eats 3 meals/day plus several snacks.

Seven Year Old
— **Movement:** motor control has improved, but it is not as important at this age. Capable of fine motor hand movements.

— **Play:** begins to prefer to play with own sex. The importance of the peer group becomes central now. Enjoys games that develop physical & mental skill. Wants more realism in play. Collects things for quantity, not quality (rocks, bottle caps, baseball cards, shells).

Parental Guidance Suggestions

— Encourage parents to visit school, talk with teacher & resolve problems. Successful school experience is critical at this age to establish positive attitudes to learning & later educational experiences.

— Note any speaking or language difficulties & seek further evaluation & necessary remediation. Confer with school authorities first.

— Provide snacks like fruit, raw vegetables, cheese, raisins, milk, & juice; have a snack shelf in refrigerator for child to help self.

— Continue to reinforce safety guides.

Common Behaviors

Enjoys illusion & magic tricks.

Likes table & card games, dominoes, checkers.

Likes books s/he can read by self; also radio, records, TV; skateboards & bicycles. Girls this age often ready also for lessons in dancing, piano, or gymnastics.

— **Socialization:** is less impulsive & boisterous in activities; quiet & reflective.

Begins to deal with the complex organization of concrete concepts; can count by 2s, 5s, & 10s; can add & subtract; can tell time, days, months, & seasons; anticipates things like Christmas, birthdays, holidays. Thinks before acting; thought is more flexible now. Begins to classify & group objects on a general level.

Cognitive conceit becomes visible. Nervous habits are common. Mutilation, body image, & castration fears develop. Wants to be like friends; competition is important.

Likes school, considers ideas of teacher important.

Eight Year Old

— **Movement:** returns to an active, vigorous phase with fine motor coordination acquired. Movements are more graceful.

— **Play:** enjoys making detailed drawings.

Reads comic books, cartoons & books (often adventure stories).

Likes board games, electronic games, craft kits, sports of all types.

Parental Guidance Suggestions

— Child will have "quiet" days & periods of shyness that need to be tolerated as part of his growing up.

May be subjected to various fears & nightmares; do not permit child to sleep with parent; reassure, comfort, but don't oversympathize or give undue attention & importance to these unless they increase in severity & frequency (then see counselor).

— Teach & set examples re: harmful use of drugs, alcohol, smoking.

— Help parents form realistic expectations of child's school achievement, development, & behavior. Parents need affirmation that child's unpredictable & changing behavior is normal & expected.

— Teach safety around autos including using seat belts, knowing rules of bike safety.

Common Behaviors

— **Socialization:** again gregarious, becomes a self-assured & pragmatic character on home ground. Eager to absorb the world around him & render opinions on all matters. Curiosity is boundless; able to collect & classify objects in a qualitative manner now.
Increasingly modest about own body. Strongly prefers the company of own sex, is selective in choice of company & likes group projects, clubs, & outings. Uses language as a tool; likes riddles, jokes, & word games; has a sense of humor. Art work begins to show new perception of subjects.

— **Feeding:** needs approximately 2100 calories/day.

Nine Year Old

— **Movement:** active, constantly on the go; plays & works hard, often to the point of fatigue. Large group skills & activities predominate (swimming, other sports, dancing).
Uses tools fairly well.
Uses both hands independently.

— **Play:** peer activities dominate with strong sex differences in play choices; hopscotch, jacks, jumprope, & crafts for girls; war games, fort building, tag, & Pop Warner football for boys. Both sexes like soccer, kickball, & softball. Board games, electronic games, after-school hobbies, music & dancing lessons popular. Reading still enjoyed by many, but school-age children now thought to watch more than 20 hours television/week.

Parental Guidance Suggestions

— Needs to be considered important by adults & given small responsibilities.

— Sex conscious; requires simple explanations, honest answers.

— Avoid negative reinforcement of teasing, nailbiting, enuresis, whining, poor manners, swearing.

— Plan meal & snack times, as child is often too busy to take time for eating proper amounts with good eating habits.

— Teach safety with firearms including storing them apart from the bullets, handling them carefully, never referring to them as a toy.

— Assess health knowledge & spend time with child discussing health habits. See references.

Common Behaviors

— **Socialization:** rules become a guiding force in all aspects of life. Overly concerned with peer-imposed rules. Interested in family life, activities, & vacations, but parents are excluded from a major portion of child's life. Shows a consuming interest in how things are made; how & what makes weather, seasons; outer space, rockets, & science fiction. Much antagonism & rivalry between sexes & between siblings, leading to frequent quarrels & teasing.

Ten Year Old

— **Movement:** very active with good coordination. Marked differences in motor skills between the sexes appear, with boys surpassing girls in strength, endurance, & agility while girls may exceed in flexibility & graceful movement; training & interests are determining variables.

— **Play:** likes gangs & clubhouse with secret codes, rules & rituals; experiments in all areas.
Enjoys crafts like weaving, jewelry & leather work; singing in choral groups.
Likes mystery stories & TV.
Interested in hobbies, collections of stamps, coins, rocks, shells, beer cans, bottle caps, license plates, etc.

— **Socialization:** is happy, cooperative, casual, & relaxed; usually courteous & well-mannered with adults.

Parental Guidance Suggestions

— Lying & stealing to gain recognition or attention may become a problem. Harsh & severe punishment should be avoided; try to restrict to room or home, cancel treats; try system of rewards with charts or lists of desired behavior. Understand & accept the child as s/he is. Know playmates & parents.

— Parental guidance & support are the strongest influence on school achievement. Competitiveness in school activities may lead to difficulties for the child in handling failure. Low self-esteem is often related to learning difficulties, below average physical skills, family & neighborhood problems. An important time to seek counseling & help PRN.

— Parental involvement & commitment are needed to encourage participation of child in organized clubs, sports, & youth groups. Be willing to serve as "team parent" or helper, since most of these activities are organized & conducted by volunteer, interested parents. Parents need to understand that while child needs time alone or with friends, there is still a need to supervise & protect child from harmful companions and influences ("R" rated movies and TV problems).

— "Latchkey" children, youngsters under 12 who are "on their own" & unsupervised after school while both parents are

Common Behaviors

Has a growing capacity for thought & conceptual organization; is able to discuss problems, see other person's point of view, think about social problems & prejudices.

The peak of the gang age; companionship is more important that play activities.

Needs occasional privacy; wants independence.

Can understand transformations of state in size, shape, weight, & volume.

Has the ability to plan ahead.

— **Feeding:** needs approximately 2400 calories/day.

Eleven Year Old

— **Movement:** differences between sexes *may* become more noticeable, as girls no longer compete on an equal basis with males in *some* areas of physical strength. Manipulative skills nearly equal to those of adults. May be the start of a stormy, active period of constant activity like finger-tapping, foot-drumming, or restless leg swinging while sitting.

— **Play:** enjoys projects & working with hands in metal craft, ceramics, auto mechanics, bicycle repair, knitting & crocheting.

Likes to do jobs and run errands that will earn money, e.g., gardening & babysitting.

Very involved in sports, dancing, & talking on telephone.

Likes participation in drama (all aspects including production, stage manager, make-up, props, publicity, etc.)

May show an interest in golf, tennis, racquetball, jogging/running, water sports, & both street & ice hockey.

Parental Guidance Suggestions

working, especially need organized community programs for their wellbeing.

— Continue sex education & preparation for adolescent body changes; see references. Since peers share sexual (mis)information, be sure children are given correct facts. Become involved with the health education program at child's school.

— Encourage inactive preteens to engage in some organized, regular play or physical exercise. It is very important to establish life-long habits of regular exercise for physical & mental wellbeing.

Common Behaviors

Indoor games of choice may include arcade games, electronic games, pingpong, pool, volleyball, & basketball. Enjoys listening to popular music; wants records, tapes of favorite stars & to attend rock concerts or movies.

— **Socialization:** rebels at routines, doing homework, or household chores. Has wide mood swings with rapid changes from moodiness to cheerfulness. May cry & lose temper if hair doesn't look "perfect" before going somewhere. Begins to take daily showers, shampoos without urging, especially as s/he begins to take notice of opposite sex. Peers are very significant; "put-downs" & taunting over physical attributes, clothing, or school skills is very common. Participates actively in community, team, & school affairs. Wants unreasonable amounts of freedom to do as s/he wishes. Wants to be trusted & given responsibility; wants to earn extra money over allowance by washing cars, mowing lawns, babysitting, etc.

Boys begin to tease girls to get attention.

Hero worship is prevalent.

Can be very critical of themselves, their own work or skills. Interested in whys of health measures; beginning to understand reproduction when accurately taught.

— **Sleeping:** needs approximately 8–10 hours/night.

— **Feeding:** males need approximately 2500 calories/day; females approximately 2250 calories/day.

Parental Guidance Suggestions

— Set realistic limits that can be tolerated by both sides. Offer support & give democratic guidance as child works through feelings. Needs help channeling energy in the right direction.

— Peer influences may cause habits of smoking or drinking to start at this age. Parents need to set clear expectations & enforceable limits on preteen behavior. Help schools arrange for suitable educational materials on smoking & alcoholism by contacting local agencies of PTA & American Cancer Society. Use power of suggestion rather than dictating behavior; set good examples of moderation & moral values for children.

— Requires adequate explanations of body changes & special understanding for child that surges ahead or lags behind. Recognize that they may have a need to rebel & deprecate others.

— Since the time of menarche continues to occur at earlier ages (it is not unusual to see menstruation occur at age 11, also some pregnancies), it is important to take early-developing girls for gynecological check-ups & health counseling.

— Avoid purchasing excessive sugar snacks & junk foods.

Recommended References

Drugs: A Primer for Young People, 2nd Ed. Phoenix, AZ: Do It Now Foundation (PO Box 5115, 85010), 1976.

Enlist in the War Against Drugs, by Home Health Education Service. Nashville, TN: Southern Publishing Assn (Box 59, 37202).

"Growing Up a Little Faster—Children in Single-Parent Households," by R. Weiss. *Children Today*, May/June 1981:22–25, 36.

Listen, A Journal of Better Living, Special Drug Issue. Mountain View, CA: Pacific Press Publishing Assn (1350 Villa St, 94042), April 1981.

Parent Group Starter Kit. Silver Spring, MD: National Federation of Parents for Drug-Free Youth (PO Box 722, 20901).

Parents, Peers, and Pot, by M. Manatt. Rockville, MD: PHS, Alcohol, Drug Abuse & Mental Health Administration, Prevention Branch, Division of Resource Development (National Institute on Drug Abuse, 5600 Fishers Lane, 20857).

The Perils of Puberty, by S. Tepper. Denver, CO: RMPP Publication (1852 Vine St, 80206).

"The Reluctant Learner: A Strategy for Intervention," by T. Millar. *Children Today*, September/October 1980:13–15.

What Every Kid Should Know, by J. Kalb and D. Viscott. Boston: Houghton Mifflin, 1976.

Normal Growth & Development: Adolescent

Definition: Adolescence spans the developmental period terminating childhood, from 12 through 19 years of age.

LONG TERM GOAL: Through this period of turmoil and rapid change, the individual will achieve social, emotional, and physical maturity as a healthy young adult; the adolescent will demonstrate an appreciation of, and security in, his own uniqueness, abilities, limits, values, feelings, and responsibility for his own behavior.

General Considerations:
— **Developmental task** (Erikson's central problem) to be resolved in adolescence is *identity* versus *identity diffusion*, i.e., who am I really? who do I want to be? and how am I different from others? During this period the adolescent continues to develop a self-concept and identity that is acceptable to oneself and one's significant others. To this end s/he "tries on" many different roles in deciding what career, role, and personality characteristics are most desirable.
— **Acceptance** is a critical element in the adolescent's pursuit for a self-concept; conformity of dress, eating, activities, appearance, and beliefs are all part of his attempts at acceptance among his peers.
— The overriding peer importance of the last period of the middle years of childhood takes on a different character during adolescence as peer groups are no longer restricted exclusively to one sex, but the individual has significant peer relationships in groups of both sexes serving different needs.
— The all-consuming importance of rules for the school age child gives way *to a severe criticism of authority and rule and a desire to change the world*, making it a better place to live. To this end the adolescent joins activist groups and civic change groups to make a contribution and effort at achieving his high goals for mankind.
— **Stress-related disorders** in adolescents (anxiety and phobic reactions, eating disorders, depression, alcohol and drug abuse, suicidal and delinquent behaviors) are more prevalent today than in previous generations due to increased social pressure and expectations of peers vs. parents. Teenagers often need help to learn that everyone has problems/conflicts/tensions, that help is available from caring others, that s/he can successfully face own feelings, understand and accept self, and that by developing stress management skills, s/he will be able to cope effectively with own problems.
— More than 12 million teenagers are sexually active beginning, on the average, about age 16 (Guttmacher Institute Report; see references). While use of contraception is increasing, more than 1 million teenage girls get pregnant each year. About three-quarters of these pregnancies are unintended. Studies show teenagers to be seriously misinformed on basic sex education facts. More than two-thirds never practice contraception, or do so inconsistently. Nearly one-half the sexually active teenage females think they

can't get pregnant, yet one-fifth of teenage pregnancies occur within the first month after start of intercourse; one-half the pregnancies occur within the first six months. Studies show that peers and the media (movies & TV) are the primary source of adolescent sex education. While over 75% of Americans favor sex education in schools, only three states and the District of Columbia require it; only seven more states encourage it. Less than one-quarter of teenage students receive a significant amount of school-based sex education. A heightened awareness and concern among the public, along with a strong commitment, may help correct this growing problem. The health professions, particularly nursing, can play a major role in providing appropriate sex education programs for youth.

— Adolescence is a special period of childhood where the individual undergoes numerous physical and emotional changes to develop into the unique individual s/he has been maturing into throughout childhood. Due to the uniqueness of each individual, it becomes difficult to set rigid standards for patterns of development, yet there is a sequential progression of behaviors during this period.

— The **common parameters** of physical development and the broad changes in behaviors for the adolescent are outlined below with corresponding nursing implications and teaching or guidance suggestions.

Twelve through Nineteen Years

Physical Development

— **Weight:**

Females	11–14 years:	101 lbs (46 kg)
	15–19 years:	120 lbs (55 kg)
Males	11–14 years:	99 lbs (45 kg)
	15–18 years:	145 lbs (66 kg)
	19 years:	147 lbs (67 kg)

— **Height:**

Females	11–14 years:	62" (157 cm)
	15–19 years:	64" (163 cm)
Males	11–14 years:	62" (157 cm)
	15–18 years:	69" (176 cm)
	19 years:	70" (178 cm)

Nursing Implications and Parental Guidance Suggestions

— Intensifed weight gain, growth spurts, & episodes of fatigue accompany adolescent physiological changes; patient, supportive counseling is needed to bolster self-confidence & encourage sound dietary practices & hygiene.

— A wide degree of variability must be allowed due to individual differences.

— Scoliosis screening should be done & referrals made as needed.

Physical Development

— **Pulse:** 50–100/minute. **Respirations:** 15–24 minute

— **BP:** 110–118/65–74

— **Teeth:** wisdom teeth usually come in, if at all, by 18–20 years average.

— **Sex Characteristics:**
Female—primary: increase in size of internal & external genitalia; changes in endometrial lining & vaginal secretions; ovulation & menarche (12–13 years average age of onset)
Secondary: increase in breast size, bone growth, BMR; changes in shape of female pelvis, pubic & axillary hair patterns; increased fat deposits in breasts, buttocks, & thighs; increasingly smooth & soft skin.
Male—primary: growth & development of testes, scrotum, & penis; production of mature sperm.
Secondary: changes in body hair distribution; increase in size of vocal cords; increased thickness of skin, sebaceous secretions, BMR, & bone growth with broadening of shoulders.

Nursing Implications and Parental Guidance Suggestions

— Caries common during this period; arrange at least twice yearly dental check-ups; screen for orthodontic problems.

— Questions & curiosity regarding the physical changes in their systems must be answered with honest & direct answers to prevent misconceptions & to foster a positive self-image. Listen sympathetically to expression of feelings (worries, fears) re: changes.

— Dysmenorrhea can be helped with anti-prostaglandin preparations (Motrin, Ponstel, Anaprox). They should be taken at the onset of menstrual period & stopped as the flow subsides. They are also useful for decreasing heavy bleeding, but not shortening the period. They should be taken with milk or food, but not with aspirin or any other medication.
Caution teenagers not to take each others' prescriptions. Each girl should be examined by a competent MD to evaluate whether cause of the dysmenorrhea is primary or secondary to some organic problem, infection, or tumor. For mild cramping, the MD may recommend two aspirin Q4H or a preparation containing a diuretic & a mild sedative. Some studies suggest that the "craving" for chocolate prior to a menstrual period is a body need for magnesium.

Physical Development

Nursing Implications and Parental Guidance Suggestions

Teach girls to use sanitary pads or tampons (regular-size only), & to change them at least twice daily. Caution against use of tampons when girl is being treated for any pelvic inflammatory disease or other illness.

If girls have been raised in families comfortable with occasional discussions of growth & sex, the beginning of menstruation will be accepted naturally with little embarrassment or tension. Teasing & dire predictions are out of place. Since myths & misinformation still abound, it is important to have an open discussion about the process, encouraging questions, beliefs, & feelings to be shared. Simply dropping a book on the subject in the girl's hands is unwise, unless requested or read together by mother & daughter. The action of giving the child something to read can be interpreted as uncaring, unwillingness, or inability on the part of the mother to discuss such private subjects. Providing clear, concise, accurate information about menstruation in a matter-of-fact way will enable the girl to reject nonsensical information shared among her friends. Assure girls that usually they can continue with normal activities, that discomfort is often only temporary, & that their periods may be very irregular for a year or more.

— Skin care is especially important; teach youth to cleanse face thoroughly with a mild, unscented soap; rinse; apply a 5 or 10% benzyl peroxide gel 1–2 x daily for pimple prevention as well as treatment; use noncomedogenic cosmetics. See Recommended References.

Twelve to Fifteen Years

Common Behaviors

Twelve to Fifteen Years

— **Movement:** often awkward & uncoordinated, as the adolescent adjusts to physical changes in height & size. Frequently displays poor posture. Physically *active*, but tires easily.

— **Leisure/Play:** enjoys activities centered around group (usually same sex, gradually mixing at social & sporting events). Enjoys school-related events (sports, dances, concerts, rallies, parties, plays, & various competitions).
Girls like shopping, talking on telephone, listening to music, spending time on make-up, hair styling, manicures, sun bathing, watching soap operas & other TV, movies, cooking, sewing, reading popular magazines, & baby sitting.
Boys enjoy listening to music, reading popular magazines, watching or participating in sports activities, working on bikes, cars, motorscooters, or other mechanical interests, watching movies & TV, playing arcade electronic games.
Both want free time, unsupervised by adults, to "do their own thing."
Both show interest in getting part-time jobs for extra spending money over regular allowances.

Parental Guidance Suggestions

— The adolescent needs reassurance & help in accepting his changing body; parents need to reinforce positive qualities, seek professional help for problems of skin eruptions, vaginal discharge, dental caries, drug use, etc.

— Set realistic but firm limits that can be mutually agreed upon for security reasons; avoid threats.

— Exercise authority with tact.

— Provide opportunities for child to earn money & have some financial independence.

— Encourage independence & allow person to be an individual, to feel s/he has some control over what happens to him; however, be available & allow child to utilize parent, as s/he needs to do so.

— Provide honest answers to questions; repeat explanations PRN.

Common Behaviors

— **Socialization:** has an increasing interest in the opposite sex. "Going around" (liking each other but not really dating yet) progresses to group dates, then couple dating alone.
Peer-group acceptance is strongest in early adolescence & the pressure to conform to group norms is nearly overwhelming to many teens.
Strong friendship bonds are formed with 1 or 2 close peers. Shows increasing hostility & alienation towards parents or authority figures. Expresses strong opinions & beliefs contrary to those of parents & school staff. Verbal conflicts over restrictions are common.
Concerned with morality, ethics, religion, & social customs; is in the process of developing own values & standards, but peer group beliefs are strong influences. Idealism is prevalent. Reasoning is mature; thinking now includes abstract ideas. Wide variations in academic abilities & interests.
Day-dreaming & sexual fantasies are common.
Girls are more socially adept than boys; will take initiative to telephone boys & plan parties or other group activities.
In early adolescence (age 12), girls have more interest than boys in physical appearance, physical development & attractiveness. By age 14, both sexes worry & fret over hair, skin, size of body parts, clothing, & physical details. As interest in opposite sex grows, so does the frequency of showers, shampoos, teeth brushing, & grooming habits.

Parental Guidance Suggestions

— Provide gentle encouragement & guidance regarding dating; avoid strong pressures of either extreme.

— Age varies on dating, as some do not date a single person until late adolescence.

— Continue to provide teenagers a warm, affectionate, loving, parental relationship. *Tell* your children you love them; tell them they are attractive, interesting, worthwhile, & special; encourage positive mental attitudes; show them respect by helping to build their self-confidence & self-esteem; praise often, criticize less. Explain that feelings do not have to be denied; that it is normal to have varied & changing moods & feelings (anger, irritability, tenderness, sensitivity, romantic longings, jealousy, guilt, anxiety, fear, embarrassment, etc.) Help them to get in touch with their feelings by talking about it with a trusted other, family member, or good friend. Parents need to understand child's conflicts as s/he attempts to deal with social, moral, political, & intellectual issues.

— Avoid increasing the levels of guilt & anxiety about masturbation by letting the adolescent know it's "OK."

— Provide information & counseling re: venereal disease, professional birth control resources. Encourage open discussion of problems, concerns, & questions. Seek family counseling for coping with an adolescent who has problems of drug abuse, pregnancy, depression, learning handicaps, or other difficulties. Consider joining a parent support group to cope with parental feelings of guilt, fear, anger, & hopelessness.

Common Behaviors
— **Sleeping:** approximately 7–9 hours/night.

— **Eating:** prefers easy-to-obtain junk foods such as candy, carbonated drinks, potato chips. Concern over appearance may lead to crash diets, poor eating patterns, or serious eating disorders.
Females need approximately 1500–3000 calories/day (average 2200/day).
Males need approximately 2000–3700 calories/day (average 2700/day)

Parental Guidance Suggestions

— Vitamin & iron supplements are often recommended.

Sixteen through Nineteen Years

Common Behaviors
— **Movement:** has increased energy as growth spurt tapers. Muscular ability & coordination increase.
— **Leisure/Play:** enjoys working for altruistic causes. Sports activities (as both participant & observer) are well-attended. Likes beach & recreational activities like surfing, skiing, sailing, tennis, volleyball, hiking. Reading, TV, music, radio, & telephone are all still important.
 Likes challenging games like chess, bridge, poker, crossword puzzles, etc.
May explore new interests via volunteer work, summer jobs, high school occupational programs, part-time employment, & vacation trips.
Dancing is popular; also enjoys attending concerts, plays, etc.
Enjoys high risk, competitive sports such as car racing.

Parental Guidance Suggestions
— Set goals with your teenagers & help them develop independence & competence in such things as grocery shopping, preparing nutritionally balanced meals, checkbook management, home & yard maintenance, first aid, health & safety measures.
— Arrange for driver education.

Common Behaviors

— **Socialization:** continues to refine language, reasoning, thinking, & communicating skills. Begins to realize that inadequacies in these areas adversely affect job opportunities & limit career choices.

Has achieved a more mature, interdependent relationship with parents. At 15 or 16, confides more in friends than in parents; at 18 or 19, parental advice & support is sought & the transition to adulthood is made.

Dating in pairs & groups is common; romantic love affairs develop. Some look for permanence in a relationship; others decide to postpone permanent relationships until completion of college or establishment of job security.

Has an increased ability to balance responsibility with pleasure. Develops an identity for self & an image of the kind of person s/he will become. Tries to develop characteristics thought to be desirable in a mate. Learns through satisfactions & frustrations of the problems living full time with peers, either in college or apartment settings. Peer group affiliation is not as rigid. Despite continuing peer influence, independent judgment emerges.

Constantly seeks satisfactory part-time jobs to pay for car, dating, & other personal expenses. Effort is directed to become independent & self-supportive. Summers are spent working or getting extra course work for college. Plans more realistically for career. Assumes major responsibility for deciding on post-high school plans. More females are now

Parental Guidance Suggestions

— Provide assistance as needed & desired for selecting a college, obtaining a scholarship & financial assistance, getting a job, planning a wedding, buying a car, getting insurance or a loan, using an acceptable, appropriate birth control method, resolving a health problem, etc.

— Parents may need help adjusting to the loss of their dependent child.

Common Behaviors

seeking educational majors & careers that were formerly dominated by males (e.g., engineering, business, medicine).

— **Sleeping:** 6–8 hours/night.

— **Eating:** females need approximately 1200–3000 calories/day (average 2100/day).
Males need approximately 2100–3900 calories/day (average 2800/day).

Parental Guidance Suggestions

— Continue vitamin & iron supplements as recommended.

Recommended References

Acne a Treatable Disease and Let's Talk Cosmetics, by J. Fulton, Jr. Newport Beach, CA: Acne Health Care Center (1587 Monrovia Avenue, 92663).

"Acne: New Approaches to an Old Problem." Consumer Reports, August 1981:472–477.

"Asking for What you Want (and Improving Your Chances of Getting It)", by J. Marks. *Teen*, June 1982:14, 18, 19, 78.

Almost Grown: A Christian Guide for Parents of Teenagers, by J. Oraker. San Francisco: Harper & Row, 1980.

"Changing Roles and You: Your Options for the Future," by J. Marks. *Teen*, February 1982:8, 9, 78.

"Counseling Sexually Active Very Young Adolescent Girls," by E. Peach. *MCN: The American Journal of Maternal Child Nursing*, May/June 1980:191–195.

How to Talk to Your Teenagers About Something That's not Easy to Talk About—Facts About the Facts of Life and *What Teens Want to Know but Don't Know How to Ask*. New York: Planned Parenthood Federation of America, Inc., (810 Seventh Ave, 10019) 1980.

Living with Teenagers, by J. and V. Rosenbaum. New York: Stein & Day, 1980.

"Medical Alert: An End to Menstrual Cramps," by M. Bechemin. *Teen*, February 1982:22–24.

Preparing for Adolescence, by J. Dobson. New York: Bantam, 1978. (Cassette Tape Album of book topics available from One Way Library, PO Box 15163, Santa Ana, CA 92705.)

"Sex Ed at the 'Y': New Approaches to a Not-So-New Problem." by J. Quinn. *Children Today*, May/June 1981:18–21, 36.

Survival Kit for Parents of Teenagers, by D. Melton. New York: St. Martins Press, 1979.

"The Teenage Mother." *NCP Guide # 4:33*, 2nd Ed., Nurseco, 1983.

Teenage Pregnancy: The Problem That Hasn't Gone Away. New York: The Alan Guttmacher Institute (360 Park Avenue S, 10010), 1981.

"What is a Normal Adolescent?" by B. Nelms. *MCN: The American Journal of Maternal Child Nursing*, November/December 1981:402–406.

The Normal Neonate

Definition: The "normal" neonate is a full term newborn infant of 38 to 42 weeks of age, weighing at least 2500 grams (5.5 lbs), with an APGAR score of 7–10, and with no abnormalities, injuries, or need of special procedures. This group excludes small for gestational age (SGA) and large for gestational age (LGA) newborns who are either less than the tenth percentile or greater than the ninetieth percentile in weight.

LONG TERM GOAL: The normal neonate will function adaptively to extra-uterine existence as a new member of a family without complications or problems that have not been promptly identified and appropriately corrected.

General Considerations:
— Review NCPG #3:22, "Normal Growth & Development: Neonate."
— **Nursing responsibilities** include:
  1) *observing, assessing*, and *recording* infant's condition within the first 12 hours of birth and regularly as condition indicates until discharge;
  2) *providing* a safe, nurturing environment;
  3) *supporting* the neonate's adjustment to life outside mother's womb;
  4) *promoting* a healthy parent-child relationship;
  5) *teaching* parents optimal care of newborn, along with appropriate expectations of normal growth and development; and
  6) *providing* family with community health nurse referral PRN.

Specific Considerations, Potential Patient Outcomes, and Nursing Actions:
1) Physical Assessment   The newborn will have abnormalities promptly and correctly identified; the newborn will be identified as a unique individual with specific characteristics; a baseline of information for subsequent exams will be established:
  — refer to NCPG #3:22, "Growth & Development: Neonate;"
  — observe & record the following parameters upon admission to nursery & daily:
    1) vital signs (TPR, BP, heart rate & rhythm), wt (grams & pounds), length (cm & inches), head circumference;
    2) appearance & condition of:
      • fontanels, head, scalp
      • eyes, ears, nose, mouth, lips, tongue, palate, & amount of mucus

- skin color, turgor, condition, marks, & presence of creases on soles of feet (not to be confused with wrinkles on feet, which occur after 24 hours of age)
- neck, trunk, limbs, & phalanges (check flexion of neck, wrist, & ankle as well as heel-to-ear & scarf sign); check for full range of motion of all limbs
- resting posture
- chest, abdomen, breasts, & genitalia
- back, spine, & anus
- cord (presence of oozing);

3) reflexes & responses to environmental stimuli: Moro, blinking, rooting, sucking, tonic neck, grasp, walking, dance, & Babinski;

4) presence, character, & frequency of voiding & stools;

5) presence, character, & frequency of "spitting-up", regurgitation, or vomiting;

6) activity pattern (quiet or active sleep; relaxed, inactive or alert, active waking periods); observe & note any tremors, seizures, or atypical movement;

7) cry-character, frequency;

8) blood glucose level, as determined by Dextrostix & heel-prick blood sample;

— check information about complications of pregnancy, labor, or delivery that might adversely affect the neonate's health status or cause development problems, including clinical assessment of gestational age;

— check to see that ID bracelet is correct & secure, that footprints & mother's thumb prints are properly recorded & not smeared;

— be sure to weigh daily at the same time on the same scale, nude, & prior to feeding.

2) Respiratory Function

The newborn will maintain an open, clear airway; the newborn will breath without difficulty and will be adequately oxygenated:

— observe, report, & record cyanosis, pallor, choking, grunting, nasal flaring, retraction, shallow or irregular respirations, poor chest expansion, & respiration rates below 35 or above 50/minute, & periods of apnea greater than 10 seconds;

— after first checking heart rate, suction oropharynx, nares, nasopharynx PRN to remove mucus; always suction mouth first as newborns are obligatory nose breathers; after suctioning, stimulate infant by rubbing soles of feet to reinforce sensory input; avoid vigorous or traumatic stimulation, so as not to stimulate vagal reflex, thereby producing bradycardia;

— keep bulb syringe or De Lee mucous trap in crib readily accessible; have mechanical suction equipment, sterile Y-connectors, & French whistle-tip catheters on hand; have oxygen & resuscitation equipment readily available & in good working order;

— position on side & change to opposite side QH; may elevate foot of bassinet from 15° to 30° to promote gravity drainage; know that position should be flat & prone if there has been a difficult passage of head or forceps delivery;

— keep infant dry & warm to prevent chilling & stressing infant, since the latter produces increased respiratory rate to compensate.

3) Nutrition   The newborn will demonstrate pronounced rooting behavior, a strong effective grasp of nipple, satisfactory sucking response, and sufficient swallowing behavior for adequate nourishment to gain weight and strength; the parent-newborn feeding pattern will be successfully and satisfactorily established:

— observe & record infant's feeding behavior readiness: presence & strength of reflexes (rooting, sucking, swallowing, gag), level of arousal when hungry, ease in burping & pattern of regurgitation; explain & demonstrate these behaviors to both parents;

— stimulate & nurture a happy, satisfying feeding time for both newborn & parent by showing parent how to hold, feed, & burp newborn successfully; by observing relationship & activity; and by providing positive feedback & encouragement to strengthen behaviors that are nurturing, comforting, satisfying, & consistently effective;

— teach both parents the what & how of prescribed formula preparation; provide written instructions & literature; encourage questions;

— *support* parent's decision to feed via breast or bottle & provide information as needed or requested; take time to explore feelings parent may have about decision, but do not be trapped into expressing an opinion to "reassure," convince, or persuade a dubious parent;

— bring breastfed babies to the mother shortly after delivery (first 4 hours) to establish feeding pattern, to stimulate milk production, & to provide newborn with antibodies in colostrum; provide breastfed babies with frequent & on-demand feedings instead of supplementary bottle feedings, which dull appetite & diminish sucking strength; if supplementary feedings are essential, give by dropper or teaspoon;

— refer PRN to NCPG #4:30, "The Mother Who Breastfeeds Her Infant."

4) Temperature

The newborn will maintain a normal body temperature in a regulated environment:
- prevent exposure & chilling by keeping newborn snugly wrapped in a lightweight blanket & by accomplishing all care & treatments quickly in a draft-free, warm environment;
- maintain nursery & mother's room temperatures within recommended range of 72–76°F, with humidity controlled at approximately 40–60%;
- postpone bathing at least 4–6 hours after birth until newborn temp reaches 36.2°C rectally; provide extra warmth until body temp stabilizes;
- prevent overheating because sweating does not occur to lower body temperature.

5) Infection Control

The newborn will have a normal drying cord and clean normal skin; the newborn will be free from infection:
- employ your hospital's standard nursery infection control procedures;
- scrub hands for 3 minutes in disinfectant solution before entering nursery environment; wash hands for at least 15 seconds before & after handling each infant;
- to prevent & control infectious agents, consider practice of cohorting (grouping in one room all neonates born within a 24–48 hour period, assigning nursing personnel to one cohort room, cleaning room throughly before admitting a new group);
- keep infants in isolated separate rooms when an airborne organism is known to be causing infection problem;
- if unable to divide staff between infected & uninfected neonates, then enforce practice of caring first for non-infected infants *before* moving on to infected infants;
- screen personnel for carrier status during outbreaks of staphylococcus or streptococcus infections;
- exclude nursing staff from nursery duty during all illnesses, especially febrile episodes, gastroenteritis, respiratory tract infections, skin infections, & active herpes simplex virus (oral or genital);
- avoid overcrowding neonates (bassinets should be at least 3 feet apart); do not increase nurse-to-patient ratio (if it can be avoided) since this increases risk of cross-contamination;
- cleanse cord & umbilicus with alcohol daily & PRN to keep clean & dry; leave exposed to air or apply dry, sterile dressing; know that bacitracin ointment may be used prophylactically; keep diaper folded below umbilicus until healing occurs;
- prevent scratching of face by trimming nails with blunt baby nail scissors; fold cuffs of long-sleeved shirt over hands when sleeping;

    — after temp has stabilized, cleanse only soiled, bloody portions of newborn skin with sterile cotton balls & sterile water; only if permitted, use mild, non-medicated soap on grossly soiled areas & rinse thoroughly; cleanse buttocks area with each diaper change, applying white petroleum jelly, hydrogenated vegetable shortening, prescriptive cream or ointment as indicated to protect from moisture, rashes, & skin breakdown;

    — within 1 hour of birth (if not previously done in delivery room), use prophylactic drug per State law in newborn eyes; do not rinse eyes, but pat dry excess solution on lids to prevent discoloration, which (if occurring) should be explained to parent as to cause & temporary nature;

    — discard & do not reuse formulas once feeding is finished;

    — do not hold newborn close to face or kiss;

    — teach parents normal hygienic practices re: handwashing before care, providing a clean environment for baby, providing proper cord care, circumcision care, & skin care following diaper changes, protecting baby from others with colds or infections, safe formula preparation (if not breastfeeding or using commercially prepared formulas), & the signs of illness to be immediately reported to to MD.

6) Prevention of Injury

The newborn will remain free of injury:

    — demonstrate, observe, & teach safe handling techniques to all who handle newborn (firm support to all body parts especially head, keeping a controlling hand on infant while weighing or giving care on any surface without protective sides or straps, placing a hand between skin & diaper when pins are used, transporting in a careful, guarded position);

    — observe & maintain safe environment, e.g., well lit, clutter-free, dry non-slip floors, approved & working electrical appliances, cribs, rocking chairs, & scales in good repair.

7) Parent-Infant Bonding

The newborn and its parents will display attachment behaviors; the parents will express an understanding of the bonding process:

    — promote rooming-in practices & father-visiting policies that encourage more opportunities for both parents to cue in to their infant: gazing, talking to, stroking, cuddling, & fondling as desired;

    — describe the positive characteristics of the infant to both parents; inform parents of infant's activity & progress frequently throughout day;

    — praise parents for appropriate parenting skills, safe handling of infant, kinds of questions asked about baby, willingness to learn baby care;

— explain the bonding process, its gradual development, & the role of reciprocal interaction;
— teach the parents appropriate growth & development expectations & how to provide a stimulating environment to foster development;
— refer to NCPG #4:32, "Parent-Infant Bonding", for additional information & nursing actions.

Discharge Planning and Teaching Objectives/Outcomes

1) (The Parents/Significant Other) Express reasonable confidence in and demonstrate successfully the ability to bathe and diaper newborn, to hold and feed baby in a reciprocally satisfying relationship, and to protect infant from injury.
2) Have written instructions for making formula and express confidence and understanding re: its correct preparation. (This includes mothers who are breastfeeding but wish to have knowledge in case of sudden need.)
3) If breastfeeding, mother has written instructions for care of breasts and descriptive literature for additional help.
4) Have referral phone numbers (community health nurse and pediatrician) for use and an appointment slip (date, time, place) for baby's first check-up.
5) Have referral information for support groups such as La Leche, Mothers of Twins Club, teenage mothers, Parents Without Partners, new mothers' groups as needed.
6) Have list of emergency services available in community.
7) Have identification bands (mother and baby) still in place and correctly matched on discharge.
8) Have an infant auto seat that meets federal safety standards.

Recommended References

"Blood Pressure Monitoring in Neonates," by N. Haddock. *MCN: The American Journal of Maternal Child Nursing*, March/April 1980:131–135.

"Caring For Your Baby," "The Mother and the Baby," and other literature. Columbus, OH: Ross Laboratories Creative Services and Information Dept. (625 N. Cleveland Ave., 43216).

"Determining A Newborn's Gestational Age," by R. Sullivan et al. *MCN: The American Journal of Maternal Child Nursing*, January/February 1979:38–45.

"Normal Growth & Development: Neonate." *NCP Guide #3:22*, 2nd Ed., Nurseco, 1983.

"Normal Newborn Care," by S. Shipman & D. Robinson, in *Protocols For Perinatal Nursing Practice*, Rosanne H. Perez, Ed. St. Louis, MO: Mosby 1981.

"Parent-Infant Bonding." *NCP Guide #4:32*, 2nd Ed., Nurseco, 1983.

"Prevention of Infection in the Nursery," by B. Hazuka. *Nursing Clinics of North America*, December 1980:825–831.

The Womanly Art of Breastfeeding, Nursing Your Baby, and other literature. Franklin Park, IL: La Leche International, Inc., (9616 Minneapolis Avenue, 60131).

The Normal Postpartum Patient

Definition: The "normal" postpartum patient is usually a happily married (self-defined) mother who has had good prenatal care; has no history of Rh factor, toxemia, disability, drug ingestion, or complicating disease during pregnancy; is between 20 and 39 years of age; and experienced an uncomplicated labor and delivery of a healthy infant, who is wanted and will be loved.

LONG TERM GOAL: The normal postpartum patient will experience a safe, comfortable, satisfying outcome for herself, spouse, and baby; she will assume parental role and responsibilities with satisfaction and a minimum of tolerable tension; she will complete the bio/psycho/social process of involution and restoration free of preventable complications.

General Considerations:

— Postpartum is that period of time, usually several weeks, between the termination of labor and the return of the reproductive tract to its normal nonpregnant state. Also called the *puerperium*, it is a vulnerable period of recovery and stabilization for family (mother, father, infant, siblings, and grandparents). Rapid physical, psychological, and emotional changes in a very short time span are energy-draining and produce a "future shock" situation abundant with strained relationships, negative feelings, and role disturbances even in the most "normal," healthy family.

— **Nursing responsibilities** must be instituted without delay since hospitalization post delivery is often *less than 36 hours*. They include supporting the bio/psycho/social process of involution and recovery, preventing complications and providing comfort; helping parents internalize the reality of their labor and delivery experience in order to proceed toward successful parent-child attachment; and facilitating a harmonious family integration and adaptation that will be mutually supportive in the months ahead.

Specific Considerations, Potential Patient Outcomes, and Nursing Actions:

1) Prevention of Complications
The patient will have a normally contracted uterus, normal lochia, and a healing perineum; the patient will give own perineal care as soon as able; the patient will be afebrile, free of infection, hemorrhage, or other preventable complications:

— check vital signs as ordered, reporting significant changes (BP should be above 90/60, P between 60–90, temp below 100.4° orally);

— check level & firmness of fundus Q30 minutes x 4, then QH x 2, then once a shift until discharge; record fundal consistency & fundal height (measured in fingerbreadths); massage uterus if not firm, rechecking in 15 minutes;

— check perineum, hemorrhoids, & episiotomy Q2–4H for bright red bleeding; note & record number of saturated pads per 8 hours; notify MD if more than 1 saturated pad/hour; note condition of perineal hematoma if present;

— observe & record color, odor, & amount of lochia Q15 minutes x 4, then QH x 2, then BID;

— assist pt. to provide own perineal care when able, including hand washing before & after care, warm sterile water cleansing after elimination, daily shower, proper directional cleansing, & aseptic placement of perineal pad; use a perineal heat lamp 15 minutes TID; apply topical medication if ordered; sitz baths QID may be indicated for acute discomfort;

— observe for post saddle/spinal anesthesia headaches & report if present; keep pt. flat in bed without a pillow, force fluids, apply abdominal binder, & give analgesic PRN;

— administer & record analgesics PRN for "afterpains."

2) Breast Care   The patient will experience lactation (or its suppression if not breastfeeding) with a minimum of tolerable discomfort; the patient will be free of preventable complications:

— *if not nursing*, apply breast binder or snug fitting bra; use ice packs to each breast at least 3–4 times daily; give aspirin or other prescribed analgesic PRN for breast discomfort; do not pump breasts; give medication to suppress lactation;

— *if nursing*, wash nipples with warm water to remove dried, oozing colostrum PRN; apply Vit. A & D ointment or nipple cream after nursing to lubricate & prevent cracking; relieve engorged breasts with warm, moist compresses for 20 minutes &/or by expressing milk by hand or pump methods; refer to NCPG #4:30, "The Mother Who Breastfeeds Her Infant," for breastfeeding suggestions & references; teach mother how to position infant to nipple in clockwise position around breast, so all quarters of breast are emptied (this is also helpful to prevent engorgement & to reduce nipple tenderness); caution mother to question & avoid taking any medications while breastfeeding, except vitamins & iron; urge fluids to compensate for deficit often occurring during labor & delivery;

— observe & report cracks, irritation, redness, warmth, tenderness, & temperatures above 37.5°C (99.5°F); teach pt. to observe for this after discharge, &, if occurring, to rest, avoid further breast irritation, & call MD (nursing mother should temporarily discontinue nursing & manually express milk).

3) Maintenance of Normal Body Functions (Nutrition, Elimination, Exercise, Rest/Sleep)

The patient will tolerate a regular diet and reestablish a normal pattern of elimination (voiding QS and normal stool); the patient will be ambulatory; the patient will sleep for 3–6 hours at a time and say she feels rested:

— give pt. fluids & food as desired & tolerated; give vitamins & iron as ordered; teach pt. about eating sensibly, including roughage in diet & having adequate fluids (at least 2000cc QD) after discharge;

— check voiding (amount, frequency, & appearance); watch for bladder distention Q15 minutes x 1H, then Q30 minutes until pt. first voids after delivery; notify MD if first voiding is less than 100cc & pt. remains distended; continue to observe for bladder distention or discomfort at least once each shift; attempt to stimulate spontaneous voiding with usual nursing practices, catheterizing only if necessary & ordered; record observations & nursing interventions;

— check bowel movements; give suppository, laxative, or enema as ordered & needed; teach pt. to wipe in a backward direction from vagina, using facial tissues or very soft toilet tissue;

— help pt. to get up to bathroom & chair first time after delivery; ambulate as soon as possible after 4 hours post delivery;

— encourage ambulation before naps, before feeding baby, & before night-time sleep; help pt. to relax muscles; give PRN medication for discomfort & sleep; try to avoid disturbing pt. so needs for rest can be adequately met; inquire & record how pt. feels after sleep; know that sleep deprivation & emotional tension of natal period can drain energy needed for recovery & resumption of roles;

— know that more than ⅔ of mothers are concerned & anxious about diet, exercise, & the return of their figure to normal; discuss feelings about postpartum figure, intentions to diet & exercise; provide a list of suggested exercises (see NCPG #3:31) with MD approval; review & demonstrate these with pt.

4) Psycho-
social
Adjustment
(to Role
Change,
Parenting
Responsi-
bilities,
Postpartum
Recovery)

The mother (and father) will express pleasure in their accomplishment of successful labor and delivery of a healthy infant; the parents will indicate acceptance and understanding of their role and responsibilities as parents by expressing realistic plans for mother and infant care during first 4–6 weeks following discharge:

— encourage mother to verbalize her feelings of labor, delivery, present condition; ask what you can do to make her more comfortable; if father participated in labor/delivery, ask him to describe his feelings & experiences;

— assess parents' adaptation to infant: do they have a name for it & call it by name? do they handle baby in a warm, cuddling manner, establishing eye contact? do they speak to baby? what is the feeling tone, manner? do they express pleasure in having baby & caring for him? if mother &/or father appear tense, look away from baby, refrain from holding it, keep asking if baby is all right, keep finding negative aspects about infant, appear unresponsive, or ask that baby be returned to nursery, explore reasons for behavior; note the behavior & ask if they could share their feelings with you; if you feel unable to listen or accept this behavior, seek consultation with parent/child nursing specialist or psychiatric/mental health nursing specialist;

— ask parents how they feel about baby after they have seen it; allow them to ventilate any disappointment regarding sex, appearance, etc.; refrain from saying "You should be thankful the baby is healthy," or any other negative admonishments; ask them about their expectations, dreams regarding a new child; compare this with reality & provide realistic feedback;

— assure parents that child is normal (if you are certain this is true) & explain what to expect in the way of growth & behavior; if this is a first child, explain natural molding of the baby's head, that it is helpful to rotate positions when putting baby down to rest, when to expect closure of fontanels (refer to NCPG #3:22, "Normal Growth & Development: Neonate"); talk about how to provide a stimulating environment to foster development;

— discuss with parents the phenomenon of "baby blues" or postpartum depression; find out what is known, believed, felt about this; explain that lack of free time & lack of cooperation from husband are two common complaints of new mothers that compound the feeling of depression, & that fatigue is also a significant & influencing factor; discuss with parents what plans have been made to prevent/relieve this, not just for the first week, but for at least for first month after delivery;

— inquire regarding the direct (physical) & moral support systems available to both parents for the first 6 weeks after discharge; what professional supports are accessible? is a referral to a community health nurse desirable?

— encourage mother to join a local mothers' support group to exchange information & to share babysitting responsibilities.

5) Parent-Infant Bonding

The parents and the newborn will participate in bonding/attachment behaviors:

— explain the bonding process, its gradual development, & the role of reciprocal interaction (refer to NCPG #4:32, "Parent-Infant Bonding);"

— promote rooming-in practices & father-visiting policies that encourage more opportunities for both parents to cue in to their infant, gazing, talking, stroking, cuddling, & fondling as desired;

— describe the positive characteristics of the infant to both parents; inform parents of infant's activity & progress frequently throughout the day;

— praise parents for appropriate parenting skills, safe handling of infant, kinds of questions asked about the baby, willingness to learn baby care;

— observe & record parent-infant interactions, responses, & progressive bonding behaviors.

Discharge Planning and Teaching Objectives/Outcomes

1) (The patient) Has written instructions re: diet, exercise, care of perineum and breasts, medications (name, purpose, dosage, etc.), birth control, and sexual relations; patient states she understands instructions and intends to comply.

2) Has participated in baby-care classes or has indicated she is knowledgeable and confident re: bathing, diapering, feeding, and essentials of newborn care (cord, circumcision, formula preparation, prevention of illness and injury); has at least one or two infant care booklets for reference.

3) Has the name and phone number of a professional health person (physician, midwife, community health nurse, licensed "baby" nurse—LVN or LPN) to call upon for assistance and guidance as desired and needed. Has referral information for support groups such as La Leche, Mothers of Twins, & other mothers' groups. Knows where infant can be taken for emergency care in her community.

4) Has postpartum check-up appointment slip (date, time, place).

Recommended References
Becoming a Parent (1978), *Mother and Baby Care at Home* (1979) and other literature. Columbus, OH: Ross Laboratories (625 N. Cleveland Ave., 43216).
"Beyond Maternity: Postpartum Concerns of Mothers," by M. Gruis. *MCN: The American Journal of Maternal Child Nursing*, May/June 1977:182–188.
"Comprehensive Care During the Postpartum Period," by C. McKenzie et al. *Nursing Clinics of North America*, March 1982:23–48.
"Family-Centered Discharge Planning Classes . . . Postpartum Instruction," by S. Austin. *MCN: The American Journal of Maternal Child Nursing*, March/April 1980:96, 97.
"The Mother Who Breastfeeds Her Infant." *NCP Guide #4:30*, 2nd Ed., Nurseco, 1983.
"Normal Growth & Development: Neonate." *NCP Guide #3:22*, 2nd Ed., Nurseco, 1983.
"The Normal Neonate." *NCP Guide #3:27*, 2nd Ed., Nurseco, 1983.
"Parent-Infant Bonding." *NCP Guide #4:32*, 2nd Ed., Nurseco, 1983.
Patient Care Plan: Vaginal Delivery—Postpartum. Chicago: The Nurses Association of the American College of Obstetricians and Gynecologists (1 E. Wacker Dr., 60611), 1978.
"She's a Multip . . . She Knows the Ropes," by R. Mercer. *MCN: The American Journal of Maternal Child Nursing*, September/October 1979:301–305.
The Womanly Art of Breastfeeding, 3rd Ed., *Nursing Your Baby*, and other literature. Franklin Park, IL: Le Leche International, Inc. (9616 Minneapolis Ave., 60131), 1981.

The Parent Experiencing Grief & Loss

LONG TERM GOAL: The parent will go through the grief and mourning process adaptively, able to cope with and talk about the loss s/he is experiencing.

General Considerations:

— Parents will go through grief and mourning when a child is stillborn, dies shortly after birth, or is deformed or abnormal in some way.

— Many nurses avoid the grieving mother because they don't know what to do; nothing they do can return the child, and they feel helpless. Nurses should know that a tangible help to the parent is to spend time with them, listening to what they say and being a good listener. Just being present, even without talking, can be comforting. Read NCPG #1:31, "Responses to Loss: The Grief and Mourning Process."

— **Nursing responsibilities** include fostering adaptive grieving, reinforcing reality, and preparing the parent(s) for returning to usual roles and responsibilities.

Specific Considerations, Potential Patient Outcomes, and Nursing Actions:

1) Over-whelming Feelings of Grief & Loss

The parent will grieve in own selected ways and will receive support from the nursing staff:

— help the parent to talk about her feelings ("Would you like to talk about what has happened?"... "What is it like for you just now?"); provide empathic listening, as this is probably the most *helpful* intervention; do not challenge her statements, but encourage her to tell you more;

— avoid platitudes like: "You're a healthy woman, you'll be able to have another child;" such statements are less than helpful, as the mother doesn't care about later, she needs to deal with "now" & her loss;

— ask the mother if she wishes to see the baby, if she has not already done so; if the baby is dead & she wishes to view the body, ask: "Have you seen a dead person before? What do you expect?" & provide information accordingly; wrapping the body in a colorful blanket & handling it tenderly & carefully will help to make the experience less horrifying for the mother;

— if the mother is ambivalent about seeing the body, discuss the pros & cons with her; tell her that other mothers who did not see their baby said later that they wished they had, that it would have been helpful (such viewing can reinforce reality & serve to cut short the "shock & disbelief" period of the grief & mourning process, a desirable situation);

— do not place the mother in a room with another mother; discuss with her ways to handle the times when the babies are out with their mothers: take a shower? close the door?
— relax & flex visiting hours to allow family/friends to visit pt. & provide needed support;
— ask the parent(s) if the baby has a name; if not, discuss the pros & cons of giving a name (many parents have said it was or would have been easier on them if they had named the baby);
— expect a variety of grief reactions & know that all are adaptive & should be supported except suicide, homicide, or other destructive reactions; anger & hostility may be projected onto the staff, to you: know that it is not meant for you personally; do not reject the pt. but rather give her support, e.g., "You must be feeling very angry right now," or, "I feel that you are really hurting inside," & continue to spend time with her;
— be prepared (by having adequate information) to discuss/take care of such things as: signing of autopsy or death certificate, what to do with the baby's clothes, possible future surgery & hospitalization for living baby;
— reassure that past deeds had nothing to do with what happened to the baby (parents sometimes blame themselves); if at all possible, make a concerted effort to find out what happened to baby & share with parent(s);
— if possible, have the same nurse each shift sit & talk with parent(s) twice/shift; allow family or friend to remain at bedside (leaving mother alone seems to intensify her grief).

2) Preparation
   for
   Discharge

The mother will begin to develop an awareness of her loss, as evidenced by asking questions about the baby:
— know that the next stage of adaptive resolution of her loss involves behaviors of asking questions about the baby, about the cause of death or deformity, and what can be done for the living child; of outbursts of crying, anger, hostility; of feeling overwhelmed, interspersed with reality;
— continue your support of her grieving process & reinforce positive, adaptive grieving; share with her the importance of allowing herself to grieve openly rather than suppressing it;
— discuss with parent(s) & family how they expect to cope when the mother goes home; assess the need for ongoing support (public health or home health nurse? referral to a mental health clinic or a private mental health worker?); provide referrals & follow up PRN; work with family so they can continue to give the parent(s) support after discharge.

Discharge Planning and Teaching Objectives/Outcomes
1) (The Parent(s)) Can talk about the loss and know that their feelings are usual, expected, and will lessen.
2) Has a resource for on-going emotional support, either in home or in a community agency, or with a private therapist.

Recommended References:
"Avoiding Communication Blocks with High Risk Parents," by S.H. Johnson. *Issues in Comprehensive Pediatric Nursing*, August 1980:61-72.
"Bereavement, the Empty-Mother Syndrome," by D.L. Wong. *MCN: The American Journal of Maternal Child Nursing*, November/December 1980:384-389.
"Bonding, Grief and Working Through In Relationship to the Congenitally Anomalous Child and His Family," by D. Vines. *Clinical and Scientific Sessions* (#NP-59). Kansas City, MO: American Nursing Association, 1979:185-192.
"Caring for the Mother of a Stillborn Baby," by T. Crout. *Nursing 80*, April 1980:70-73.
"The Child is Dying: Who Helps the Family?" by H. Williams, et al. MCN: *The American Journal of Maternal Child Nursing*, July/August 1981:261-265.
"Death of an Infant," by B. Wooten. MCN: *The American Journal of Maternal Child Nursing*, July/August 1981:257-260.
"Family Support in Infant Death," by A. Cordell et al. *JOGN Nursing*, July/August 1981:281-285.
"Having a Handicapped Child," by M. Lepler. MCN: *The American Journal of Maternal Child Nursing*, January-February 1978:32-33.
"Parents Visiting Parents For Unequal Support," by M. Eager et al. MCN: *The American Journal of Maternal Child Nursing*, January/February 1980:35-36.
"The Patient Experiencing Guilt." *NCP Guide #5:31*, Nurseco, 1981.
"Responses to Loss: the Grief and Mourning Process." *NCP Guide #1:31*, 2nd Ed., Nurseco, 1980.
"Therapeutic Groups for Parents of High Risk Infants," by J. Houser. *Issues in Comprehensive Pediatric Nursing*, August 1980:31-35.

Play Therapy: General Suggestions

Definition: Play is the natural language of a child; it is the expression of his bio/psycho/social being in relation to his environment. Therapeutic play is a supervised, semi-structured play experience that is deliberately planned, observed, and evaluated in relation to its intended objectives.

GOALS: The child will continue normal growth and development during hospitalization via play;
the child will express his ideas, feelings, and imagination through play;
the child will develop creativity through appropriate play experiences;
the child will adapt more effectively to the stress of illness/hospitalization through play; and
the child will have fun finding himself in play, given the time, materials, and opportunity.

General Considerations:

— **During hospitalization,** clinic visits, or illness experiences in the home, a child is limited in the expression of normal play outlets and opportunities. As a result, inhibition of the child's ability to grow, develop, learn, express himself, communicate, relate to his environment, and cope effectively with the stress of accident, injury, illness, loss, hospitalization, discomfort, and separation from loved ones is severely hampered. Fears are intensified, normal emotional outlets are restricted to maladaptive ones of acting out, internalization, and denial (among others), and, in addition, energy needed for healing and a return to wellness is otherwise expended.

— **Play therapy** can be used to develop the child's confidence and trust in the medical and nursing staff, to ask or answer questions and provide information in the diagnostic and treatment process, and to provide a healthy outlet for the expression of emotional responses to the stress of illness and/or hospitalization. Laughter, joy, relaxation, and enjoyment that results from appropriate play activities support the healing process and facilitate treatment.

— **Nursing responsibilities** include assessment, planning, implementation, observation, evaluation, and recording activities of play therapy to assist the child to achieve the goals listed above. In addition, the nurse should discuss with the attending physician the need for referral and psychiatric or mental health consultation, when observed play activities deviate widely from age-expected activities.

Assessment and Planning

1) Review the admission assessment, the diagnostic implications, the stage of growth and development, the nursing care plan, and the abilities of each child who is to participate in a planned play program. Prescribe individually appropriate toys, activities, and play opportunities. Clearly have in mind the purpose(s) of the play, e.g., pure pleasure, relief of anxiety, expression of creativity, the channeling of energy, distraction, explaining or teaching a diagnostic or treatment procedure, etc. Refer to NCPGs #3:23–25, "Normal Growth & Development: Infant to School-Age Child."

2) Prepare a playroom for ambulatory patients and a portable cart for bedfast patients. Consult pre-school and school age teachers, recreation specialists, parents *and children* for suggested equipment and supplies. Use *your* imagination! Some items that could be included are:

paper	plastic building blocks	egg cartons	popsicle sticks
pencils	paste	fabric scraps	empty thread spools
crayons	pipe cleaners	puzzles	tongue depressors
non-toxic marking pens	scissors	playing cards	empty toilet paper rolls
string, yarn	old magazines	games	soap solution to blow bubbles
coat hanger	balloons	clay/Play-Doh	ping pong or plastic golf balls
cellophane and paper tape	puppets	colored paper	paper or plastic drinking straws

Implementation and Evaluation

1) Have a play coordinator/specialist to conduct program, supervise volunteers, provide consultative assistance and patient behavior information to health professionals.
2) Conduct special event parties for children.
3) Use community resource volunteers for entertainment (musicians, magicians, clowns, dancers, actors, puppeteers, etc.).
4) Use tapes, records, books, and cartoon movies available on free loan from community libraries, schools, recreation centers.
5) Ask school age patients to write poems, stories, or plays about someone or something in the hospital.
6) Provide and encourage drawing, coloring, and water painting for self-expression. Avoid use of "coloring books" and structured "art."

7) Observe the play of children who present behavior problems: note child's failure to respond to age-appropriate toys and play materials, attempts at self-stimulation (rocking, head-banging, etc.), or attempts at risk-taking, dangerous, or self-destructive activities. Acknowledge feelings and encourage the child to express them verbally; convey acceptance and empathic understanding. Listen to what is revealed and not revealed. Share observations and findings with other health care professionals.

8) Record on child's chart pertinent observations re: play experiences and responses, revealed fears, feelings, and indications of new insights.

9) Obtain verbal and written evaluations of the play therapy program's success for children, parents, physicians, nurses, and others.

Recommended References

"Breathing Exercises As Play for Asthmatic Children," by H. McCaully. *MCN: The American Journal of Maternal Child Nursing*, September/October 1980:340–344.

"Communicating With Young Children" (series). *American Journal of Nursing*, December 1977:1960–1968.

"Normal Growth & Development: Infant to School Age Child." *NCP Guides #3:23–25*, 2nd Ed., Nurseco, 1983.

"Play for the Hospitalized Child," by J. Maurer. *Point of View*, January 1, 1980:4–5.

"Puppets in the Nursing Process," by M. Gustafson. *Supervisor Nurse*, November 1980:33–35.

Sesame Street Hospital Admission Kit. Milwaukee, WI: Will Ross, Inc., (Dept. AJN, PO Box 372, 4285 N. Port Washington Road, 53201).

"Use of Therapeutic Play in the Ambulatory Pediatric Hematology Clinic," by M. Taylor and H. Williams. *Cancer Nursing*, December 1980:433–437.

Postpartum Exercises

GOALS: The postpartum woman will tone and tighten the muscles of the waist, hips, thighs, and stomach; she will reduce fatty deposits that have collected.

General Considerations:

— Body reconditioning exercises for 10 minutes each day should be begun two to three weeks after delivery depending upon physician's advice.

— Teach or review with patient general principles of back care and back exercises (see NCPGs #3:41, 42). These will restore abdominal muscle strength and improve posture.

— Have patient set aside a special time each day for exercising and stick to it.

— Teach patient to breathe deeply and relax for one minute between each exercise.

— Demonstrate exercises to patient, then have her review written exercises and ask any necessary questions; suggest that she contact a nurse (friend, neighbor, or someone from a home health agency) to supervise the first time she does exercises at home.

— Teach patient always to "warm up" and "cool down" before and after exercising to prevent muscle injury. This involves four or five deep breathing and stretching exercises (#1 & #2 below).

Specific Exercises:

1) Stand with feet about 20 inches apart. Reach arms overhead toward the ceiling, rising up on tip-toes. Breathe deeply inward as you go up; hold for three seconds; then exhale while returning to starting position. Repeat 3x.

2) Lie down on back and draw both legs toward abdomen, bending knees. Stretch legs upward over hips and "bicycle ride" for 10 seconds while breathing naturally. Lower legs to floor; rest 10 seconds. Repeat 2x.

3) Lie flat on floor, legs together, arms outstretched, with a light-weight book in each hand. Breathing naturally, raise arms overhead along floor, and touch books together. Return to original position. Rest. Repeat 3–4x. (This exercise strengthens pectoral muscles and is good also for nursing mothers.)

4) While lying in supine position, tense abdominal muscles tightly and hold for 3–5 seconds. (Do *not* hold breath also at this time.) Relax. Deep breathe. Repeat 3x. In same position, squeeze perineum and rectal muscles tightly, as if to prevent involuntary elimination. Hold for 3 seconds. Relax. Repeat 3x.

5) In supine position, with arms alongside body and hands tucked underneath buttocks for support, bend knees and draw heels up to hands raising bent legs over chest, straighten legs at 90° angle to body and SLOWLY lower both legs, scissoring them back and forth while counting to eight as they are lowered to starting position. Rest. Deep breathe. Repeat 3x.

6) In a sitting position with legs straight and spread wide apart (straddle sit), reach forward with hands to grasp foot. Pull head down to knee without bending leg. Repeat on opposite leg. Then clasp hands behind neck and reach forward to touch elbows to floor between legs. Return to starting position. Relax. Breathe deeply. Repeat 3-part exercise 4x.

7) In a crawl position, with straight arms and upper legs perpendicular to floor, take a deep breath while sucking in abdomen. Bend arms touching head to floor. Exhale. Rest. Return to starting position. Repeat 3x.

8) Stand. Breathe deeply. Repeat Exercise #1. If a longer exercise period is desired, proceed through the back exercises (NCPG #3:42).

Recommended References
"Back Care." *NCP Guide # 3:41*, 2nd Ed., Nurseco, 1983.
"Back Exercises." *NCP Guide #3:42*, 2nd Ed., Nurseco, 1983.
Nursing Care of the Growing Family, 2nd Ed., by A. Pillitteri. Boston: Little Brown, 1981:397–398.
"Preventing Back Abuse in Young Mothers," by S. Cooper. *MCN: The American Journal of Maternal Child Nursing*, July/August 1977:260–263.
Rapid Post Natal Figure Recovery, by C. Reed. Raritan, NJ: (Ortho Pharmaceutical Corp., 08869).

Teaching the Parent/Guardian/Child: General Suggestions

GOAL: The parent/guardian and the child, when appropriate, will demonstrate the necessary skills, confident attitude, and essential knowledge for the effective control of the child's disease/disability and for solving the problems of daily living within unavoidable limitations.

Nursing Actions:
1) Refer to suggestions given in NCPGs #1:49, "Teaching Patients: General Suggestions," and #1:50, "Teaching Patients: Specific Plan for Skills and Procedures."
2) Refer to the discharge planning and teaching objectives of the nursing care planning guide for the condition that the child has.
3) Identify learning needs of parent/guardian/older sibling caretaker, and child, when appropriate. Assess the readiness and learning abilities of the learner(s). Include in your planning consideration of any special conditions, settings, equipment, or problems that may affect the care to be given the child.
4) Involve the learner(s) in the planning, implementation, and evaluation of the teaching program.
5) Set teaching priorities according to: (a) importance of patient/client's need (i.e., for survival or for well-being) and (b) the amount of time available.
6) Provide information that will meet the learning needs that you have identified. Use a relaxed, fairly informal manner. Keep explanations simple and teaching sessions short (about 15–30 minutes). Reduce distractions and interruptions. Allow time for thinking, absorbing new information. Encourage questions.
7) Use visual aids (films, slides, pictures, charts) when you teach, even on a one-to-one basis. Post charts and pictures on hallway walls or around a classroom for easy accessibility and frequent referral. Use bulletin board displays with changing composition and educational themes. Consider using puppets to "teach" the pre-school child and peers to teach the teenager. Use the same equipment and supplies that will be used at home. Use models such as "Ambubaby" for teaching resuscitation. Make use of your own hospital's resources: booklets, leaflets, teaching sheets.
8) Supervise return demonstrations and several successful practice sessions for skills taught.
9) Provide a means for learner to review what has been taught and to extend or share that knowledge with others at home who need to know. Consider supplying appropriate printed literature (bilingual if necessary), illustrations, diagrams, and written instructions.
10) Make referrals of the patient and family to community agencies with education services, to an ex-patient/family/support group who is successfully rehabilitated and willing to help, and/or to community health agency.

11) Chart on the patient's record all the subjects taught, to whom taught (list), the learner(s)' reaction, and an evaluation of what has been learned (results of a verbal or written test, documentation of satisfactory return demonstrations, etc.) Use the standard form of your agency if one is available.

12) Follow up to determine if your teaching was realistic, successful, and effective. Contact the community health nurse (if a referral was made), or the home care coordinator (if your hospital has one). Consider calling patient/family yourself to see how s/he is getting along.

13) After several similar teaching experiences, analyze your findings and consider possibilities of group teaching on a regularly scheduled basis. Explore feasibility of publishing booklets on commonly needed subjects, e.g., preparation for various treatments, first hospitalization, care care at home, care of tracheotomies, home care of diarrhea, other useful topics.

Recommended References

"Administering Injections to Different-Aged Children," by M. Evans and B. Hansen. *MCN: The American Journal of Maternal Child Nursing*, May/June 1981:194–199.

A Conceptual Approach to the Nursing of Children—Health Care from Birth through Adolescence, by R. Wieczorek and J. Natapoff. Philadelphia: Lippincott, 1981.

Essentials of Pediatric Nursing, by L. Whaley and D. Wong. St. Louis: Mosby, 1982.

"Preparing a Child for Procedures," by B. Hansen and M. Evans. *MCN: The American Journal of Maternal Child Nursing*, November/December 1981:392–397.

"Teaching Patients: General Suggestions." *NCP Guide #1:49*, 2nd Ed., Nurseco, 1980.

"Teaching Patients: Specific Plan for Skills and Procedures." *NCP Guide #1:50*, 2nd Ed., Nurseco, 1980.

The Aged Patient: Reality Orientation

Definition: Reality Orientation Therapy (ROT) is a group of psychosocial techniques that continually stimulate the brain to function in compensation for brain damage due to disease, injury, senility, or disuse deterioration.

LONG TERM GOAL: The patient will regain contact with reality, behaving with lessened confusion, disorientation, forgetfulness, and dependency.

General Considerations:

— **Reality Orientation Therapy** involves a program of total professional staff and visitor actions along with patient activities on a *24 hour, 7 day-a-week basis*. The earlier therapy begins after the onset of confusion, the more effective it is likely to be.

— **To cope** with the frustrations, anxiety, and depression associated with care of the senile, confused elderly patient, the *nurse must* first of all, *understand* (and appreciate the nursing *implications* associated with) the bio/psycho/social changes of *aging* as well as the environmental factors that contribute to senility and disorientation. Therefore, review the following NCP Guides: #2:33, "The Aged Patient: Physiology of Aging;" #2:26, "The Aged Patient: Common Behaviors;" and #2:27, "The Aged Patient: Transition to Communal Living."

— Although the majority of patients needing Reality Orientation Therapy are elderly, some patients will be young or middle-aged. In the latter groups, the cause of the confusion/disorientation is more likely to be related to disease, injury, drugs, or physiological and psychological abnormalities, and health care personnel are more apt to be optimistic about the patient's prognosis and more vigorously determined to alleviate cause and reverse the disorientation. Therefore, it may be necessary to re-sensitize nurses to the *importance* of a *positive attitude* and a relentless approach to helping the patient even when the patient is elderly.

— **The key to success** is consistency of expectations, attitudes, and approach on the part of staff, family, and friends. In addition, *the staff observes, reports, records, and rewards* (appropriately) even small behavioral changes that indicate progress. A weekly team conference to discuss patient progress, problems, and approaches is usually most helpful. Nevertheless, under the best circumstances, studies have shown that as many as 50% or more patients will show little or no significant change. Optimism should be tempered with realism.

— **When the patient has achieved the basic goals of ROT** (see below under patient outcomes), s/he often becomes a candidate for Educational Therapy, Resocialization and Remotivation Therapy, and Occupational Therapy. In some settings these combined therapies are referred to as Advanced Reality Orientation and are provided in a formal classroom setting with other patients. More informal but regularly scheduled and planned ''growth'' groups are another method of helping the patient become more alert, responsive, and interpersonally competent. Refer to NCPG #3:34, ''The Aged Patient: Resocialization,'' and NCPG #4:35, ''The Aged Patient: Remotivation.'' Because therapeutic effectiveness of reality orientation therapy is associated with concepts of behavior modification, refer also to NCPG #5:37, ''Behavior Modification,'' for additional information.

Specific Considerations, Potential Patient Outcomes, and Nursing Actions:

1) Sensory/ Perceptual Alterations (Deprivation Monotony, Distortion, Overload)

The patient will correctly perceive sensory stimuli, will interpret environment more accurately than before ROT; the patient will appear less withdrawn and apathetic, more alert and responsive:
— secure eye glasses, hearing aid, false teeth, & other assistive devices pt. needs for activities of daily living;
— arrange for pt. to be in an upright position, preferably walking or sitting as often as feasible; refer to NCPG #2:45, ''Hazards of Immobility;''
— provide physical exercise for pt. in a different setting, e.g., a walk, or exercises while sitting; see NCPG #2:32, ''Exercise for Patients Over 65;''
— call attention to sights, sounds, smells, taste, & interpretation of them;
— increase sensory input with flower arrangements, new taste treats, use of spices (sucking on a clove, putting spices into jars and smelling to identify, using various flavorings in tea or desserts such as mint, almond, orange, or lemon, alternatives to vanilla & chocolate);
— use music in a changing variety (e.g., marches, polkas, lyrical, restful, jazz, sing-a-long types, etc.) via tapes, radio, phonograph record; sing to pt. while giving care; arrange for music groups from local schools to give concerts for pts.;
— refer to NCPG #1:32, ''The Patient Experiencing Sensory Disturbances,'' for additional information & suggestions.

2) Impaired
Thought
Processes
(Forget-
fulness,
Short Atten-
tion Span,
Apathy)

The patient will increase his/her attention span and will concentrate for longer periods of time; the patient will correctly identify self and where s/he is; the patient will know time, day, and date with the help of clocks and calendars:
— think twice about placing a confused pt. next to a nurses station, so s/he can be more closely watched, since this
   is sometimes perceived as humiliating to the family/friends;
— plan an individualized orientation session based upon pt.'s specific needs; do not expect too much; keep goals
   attainable in small increments;
— identify previous & present reinforcers (rewards) that bring pleasure to a specific pt.; incorporate this information
   into the written care plan & utilize whenever pt. behaves in an acceptable or desired manner or gives a correct
   response;
— help reduce pt.'s frustrations by keeping questions to the easy, familiar, simple level until s/he achieves successful responses; allow sufficient time for pt. to formulate & produce an appropriate reply;
— provide clocks, calendars, & pictures of friends, family, pets, or favorite objects & interests (sports, nature,
   children, antiques); refer to these several times daily;
— always address the pt. by name, state name of hospital & day of the week; add date with month & year;
— conserve pt.'s energy for normal cognitive processes by reducing causes of fatigue (allowing short naps, alternating periods of rest & exercise or teaching);
— present facts in a friendly, kind, firm, yet matter-of-fact, simple, & clear manner; repeat, using same or different
   words ad lib;
— reinforce information with sensory aids (audio, visual, tactile, olfactory, etc.) PRN; be sure that pt. has eyeglasses
   & hearing aid PRN;
— enlist help of family, friends, housekeeping staff & others to correct pt.'s misconceptions gently & pleasantly
   without criticism;
— allow family & visitors to remain with pt. as much as possible;
— provide slow, careful, detailed information re: all tests, treatments, medications, & care activities; try to elicit a
   reaction, comment, opinion, preference, & praise any appropriate attempts to respond;

— help pt. assimilate knowledge provided by asking questions (who? what? why? when? how?); be patient, wait calmly for reply; smile & compliment pt. for repeating information accurately; if pt. cannot provide a correct answer, tell him the answer & ask him to repeat it;

— encourage pt. to ask questions of staff & to write down questions for MD; help pt. print or write as needed;

— ask pt. to identify feelings & thoughts; reflect these, encouraging elaboration;

— use TV quiz shows, radio talk shows to stimulate thought; do *not* have music playing while teaching, conversing, or trying to stimulate brain function;

— know that while the adaptive value of reminiscing has not been conclusively demonstrated, nevertheless it is considered to be beneficial for pts. who may be otherwise confused on current events & recent memories; know that having the pt. review his life *can* sometimes provide important clues about former friends & activities that brought the pt. pleasure & satisfaction, can provide opportunities to enhance the pt.'s self-concept & self-esteem, & can provide a useful means to resolve old griefs or stressful events, thereby achieving a better level of adaption to present circumstances.

3) Dependency The patient will make some decisions and choices with increased frequency; the patient will carry out some of own daily hygiene with increasing willingness and independence, requiring minimum staff supervision and assistance:

— give pt. certain kinds of control/choices; help to see how s/he can exercise this control (e.g., time or type of bath, location of chair in dayroom or dining room, type of fruit juice or food, etc.);

— promote self-care within the pt.'s known abilities & limitations; give help as needed but don't take over tasks because it is easier or more convenient for you; allow pt. plenty of time; don't hurry pt. or show impatience as it may increase the pt.'s feelings of helplessness & irritation;

— avoid IV fluids & tube feedings unless absolutely necessary;

— try to follow a set routine & assign the same care personnel as much as possible, so that consistency & comfort is experienced by pt., thereby reducing confusion;

— explain or demonstrate each new procedure slowly & repeatedly, as you assist pt. to participate actively;

— observe, report, & reward appropriately even small changes toward more independent behavior;

— refer to NCPG #1:25, "The Patient Experiencing Dependency."

Discharge Planning and Teaching Objectives/Outcomes
1) (Patient/Family/Significant Other) Has a copy of public information pamphlets or written instructions re: needs of patient for continuing reality orientation techniques.
2) Understands medical regimen and rehabilitation program, and indicates a willingness to follow it.
3) Verbalizes intent to contact physician or community health nurse for untoward signs of increasing confusion, disorientation, diminished awareness or responsiveness, and abnormal behavior.

Recommended References
"The Aged Patient: Common Behaviors." *NCP Guide #2:26*, 2nd Ed., Nurseco, 1980.
"The Aged Patient: Exercises for Patients Over 65." *NCP Guide #2:32*, 2nd Ed., Nurseco, 1980.
"The Aged Patient: Physiology of Aging." *NCP Guide #2:33*, 2nd Ed., Nurseco, 1980.
"The Aged Patient: Remotivation." *NCP Guide #4:35*, 2nd Ed., Nurseco, 1983.
"The Aged Patient: Resocialization." *NCP Guide #3:34*, 2nd Ed., Nurseco, 1983.
"The Aged Patient: Transition to Communal Living." *NCP Guide #2:27*, 2nd Ed., Nurseco, 1980.
"Behavior Modification." *NCP Guide #5:37*, Nurseco, 1981.
"Dealing with the Confused Patient," by K. Kroner. *Nursing 79*, November 1979:71-78.
"Don't Give Up! There Are Many Ways to Reach the Elderly," by D. Keyser. *Journal of Practical Nursing*, August 1980:25, 26.
"Hazards of Immobility." *NCP Guide #2:45*, 2nd Ed., Nurseco, 1980.
"Hypovigilance," by N. Meinhart and M.J. Aspinall. *American Journal of Nursing*, July 1969:994-998 (especially excellent and useful).
"I Happen To Be Older" and "Reality Orientation Goin' Home" (public information leaflets for family and friends). Arlington Heights, IL: Intercraft Associates (P.O. Box 612, 60006).
"The Patient Experiencing Confusion." *NCP Guide #1:23*, 2nd Ed., Nurseco, 1980.
"The Patient Experiencing Dependency." *NCP Guide #1:25*, 2nd Ed., Nurseco, 1980.
"The Patient Experiencing Sensory Disturbances." *NCP Guide #1:32*, 2nd Ed., Nurseco, 1980.
"Reality Orientation and Effective Reinforcement," by N. Langston. *Journal of Gerontological Nursing*, April 1981:224-227.
"Reminiscing Psychotherapy with Aging People," by K. King. *Journal of Psychosocial Nursing and Mental Health Services*, February 1982:21-25.

The Aged Patient: Resocialization

Definition: Resocialization is a type of therapy that continually stimulates the patient to interact effectively with other persons and with the social environment.

LONG TERM GOAL: The patient will be normally sociable, spending time with friends or relatives, initiating conversation, and focusing on others rather than on self.

General Considerations:
— A resocialization program of therapeutically selected activities should include only those patients in touch with reality *OR* those who have successfully participated in an intensive basic reality orientation program. Review NCPG #3:33, "The Aged Patient: Reality Orientation."
— Only those other patients in touch with reality should be permitted to interact with the patient on a one-to-one basis. In loosely structured groups of patients, at least one health care person should always be present to promote successful interaction, facilitate conversation or appropriate responses to stimuli offered.
— Patients who have successfully achieved goals of a formal resocialization program may then be suitable candidates for a more intensive rehabilitation program (occupational, educational, and vocational training), followed by a discharge preparation program.
— **Resocialization activities** should be planned with the individual's premorbid, preinstitutionalization personality, hobbies, interests, and life achievements in mind. At the same time new skills, new interests, new ideas can be successfully achieved with satisfaction by the patient when a carefully conceived, correctly and consistently implemented plan is followed by a totally involved and caring staff. Remember, however, in the zeal to employ an intensive program of resocialization for a patient, to still respect and make an effort to provide a way of meeting a patient's need for privacy, undisturbed silence, meditation, prayer, or thoughtful reflection.

Specific Considerations, Potential Patient Outcomes, and Nursing Actions:

1) Alteration in Sociali- zation (Withdrawal/ Disengage- ment, Psycho- social Isolation, Diminished Self Esteem & Confi- dence, Shyness, Embarrass- ment Loneliness, Lack of Family, Friends, or "Significant Other")

The patient will comply willingly with staff wishes that s/he seek out the company of at least one other person; the patient will demonstrate an interest in those around him and in his environment; the patient's appearance and remarks will indicate an increase in confidence and self-respect; the patient will increase communication skills, initiating conversations or single comments more frequently than before:

— if pt. is passive & compliant, discuss in matter-of-fact way the proposed social interaction, situation, or person s/he is to be with (i.e., scheduled activity, type of clothes needed, length of time it will take, behavior expected of him); try to elicit comments, expressed preferences, choices of activity or companion upon return to room or after planned social activity; reward any positive behaviors with enthusiasm, smiles, & warmth; try to elicit an expression of choice about further similar contacts;

— assess pt.'s health status, background, & past or present interests to select (or offer choices of) most desirable activities (a walk outdoors, a visit to another dept. or section of institution, a drive, a sport event, musical or dramatic production, group games, attendance at religious services, shopping expedition, etc.);

— exercise judgment to avoid excessive stimulation, fright, or discomfort caused by too many strange persons or too many activities too quickly; observe & record pt.'s reactions & adjustment to each new situation;

— introduce one new pt. or staff member at a time & allow time for getting acquainted; after a number of persons have become acquainted, then arrange for small groups to meet for some specific purpose or activity;

— prepare arrangements of wallet-sized pictures of staff members & patients with names & titles underneath; visit these charts with pts. & ask them to name each person they have met (while covering name underneath); offer special privileges or recognition to pts. who can "name them all" or have made the most progress in learning names;

— change beds or room assignments to encourage friendships, associates with mutual interests or similar backgrounds;

— provide special recognition & celebration of pt.'s birthdays or other important events & anniversaries; have other pts. join in preparation & planning of treats, surprises, gifts, decoration, entertainment, selection of music, etc.

2) Alteration in Affiliation (Lack of "Belonging-ness" or "Related-ness," Lack of Role/Involvement in a Formal, Structured Group, Lack of Object Relationships (Books, Plants, Pets, Collections, etc.))

The patient will participate in a group, listening actively, responding appropriately, offering comments, and relating with the other members; the patient will express enjoyment or pleasure in the group activity and will express regret or sadness when it is over or when s/he must miss it:

— plan formal structured group sessions of 4 to 8 pts. to perform a task, to study a topic, to develop interest or cultivate a hobby (e.g., sing-a-longs, travel, or geography groups, sports fans, gardening club, charades or dramatics, etc.);

— schedule regular times for meetings of group; limit length to 30 or 35 minutes (rarely longer because of short attention spans, need for change of positions);

— use a small room & keep group close to each other;

— serve refreshments & have pt. dress up for group meetings;

— have group leader prepare for meeting by taking time to establish a personal, trusting relationship with each member prior to inviting them to join a group; social bonding of leader to member helps pt. overcome fear of rejection & fear of attachment with anticipatory loss that are often the basis of resistance to joining a group; know that pts. may also reject a group leader that they feel will be leaving them after they become attached (e.g., a student leader on temporary assignment); know that if group leader lowers the defenses of its members— thereby making them vulnerable to the painful loss of relationships—s/he must help them develop capacity to sustain other relationships so they can reduce & offset the painful discomfort of losing their leader; help leader share own feelings of attachment & subsequent sadness with group when group experience is about to end; this will help facilitate members being able to share their feelings openly;

— allow & encourage pts. to facilitate participation by each member; reward each person's contribution; encourage members to interact with each other, not just with the leader whom they trust;

— keep membership of the group stable so that trust, openness, & role identification can take place; encourage members to shake hands, hug or kiss, welcome each other, express concern over how a member feels, etc.;

— form a reminiscing group wherein members share experiences, accomplishments, travels; as a group leader, listen attentively, express appreciation to contributing members, reinforce the value & importance of life-review reminiscing; acknowledge feelings expressed; encourage both negative & positive feelings ("It's all right to feel that way."); teach family members about the significance of reminiscing behavior & how to encourage its satisfying expression;

— consider establishing an intergenerational sharing program with local pre-schools or elementary schools whereby mutual visits can occur & friendships can develop;

— explore the feasibility of having community-based senior citizen groups meet at the health care facility for luncheons, cards, movies, concerts, or other reasons so that in-patients may attend & become involved with others in community;

— know the therapeutic value of programs & facilities that allow pet-visiting privileges & in-house animal "mascots" or birds; explore feasibility of establishing pet-oriented project in your geriatric facility;

— hold staff conferences & family conferences about the pt.'s progress, needs, social relationships; then plan to have pt. involved in these conferences to contribute own perceptions, ideas, & choices.

Discharge Planning and Teaching Objectives/Outcomes

1) (Patient/Family/Significant Other) Expresses awareness of current problems and needs and has a plan for continuing to reinforce progress made toward socialization.

2) Understands medical regimen and rehabilitation program and indicates a willingness to follow it.

3) Verbalizes intent to contact physician or community health nurse for untoward signs of apathy, boredom, loneliness, disengagement, regressed behavior, etc.

Recommended References

"The Aged Patient: Remotivation." *NCP Guide #4:35*, 2nd Ed., Nurseco, 1983.

"The Aged Patient: Reality Orientation." *NCP Guide #3:33*, 2nd Ed., Nurseco, 1983.

"Fear of Loss and Attachment," by C. Carter and D. Galliano. *Journal of Gerontological Nursing*, June 1981:342–349.

"Nursing Intervention In Support of Reminiscence," by M. Ryden. *Journal of Gerontological Nursing*, August 1981:461–463.

The Patient Experiencing Depression (Psychiatric)

Definition: Depression is an affective disorder characterized by an alteration in mood in the direction of abnormally low spirits, and accompanied by intense and sustained feelings of despondence, hopelessness, powerlessness, and emptiness.

LONG TERM GOAL: The patient will deal with painful feelings by learning to share, express, and resolve them; the patient will resume effective management of own life, as evidenced by ability to carry out activities of daily living and resume job or usual roles.

General Considerations:

— Depression is a reaction or a response to failure or loss. The word "depression" is often used to refer to "the blues" or the sadness and grief that are normal psychological responses to a loss; true depression, however, differs from "the blues" et al. in that the latter are time-limited and proportionate to what was lost. (See NCPG #1:31, "Responses to Loss: The Grief and Mourning Process.")

— There are many **views and kinds** of depression. It may be viewed as (1) *a mood state* in which the person experiences intense feelings of despair, worthlessness, gloom, emptiness, numbness, and a sense of foreboding; as (2) *a syndrome or symptom complex*: classifications within this category include agitated or retarded depression (refers to motor activity), neurotic or psychotic depression, and reactive or endogenous depression; as (3) *a disease process*, which includes manic-depressive psychosis, plus involutional, neurotic, and psychotic depression; or as (4) *a complex of psychodynamic mechanisms* (according to psychoanalytic theory), which views depression as a person's emotional expression of hopelessness and helplessness, characterized by loss of self-esteem in reaction to threatened aspirations and wishes to be loved, worthy, and appreciated; to be good, loving, and unaggressive; and to be strong, superior, and secure.

— **Neurotic and psychotic depression** have many similarities as well as some marked differences:

	Neurotic	**Psychotic**
• **Definition**	A state of depression in which *reality testing* is largely intact and *physiological disturbances*, if present, are mild.	A state of depression of psychotic intensity in which *reality testing is severely impaired*, and *physiological disturbances* (vegetative signs) *are present*.
• **Behaviors**	Sadness, melancholia, crying, withdrawal, difficulty in concentrating, anorexia, slowness of speech and move-	Marked sadness, extreme melancholia, persistent withdrawal, inability to concentrate, vegetative signs

ment, apathy, little initiative, feeling sorry for self, overt anxiety; behaviors are more severe and last longer than with "the blues" or reaction to a loss.

(anorexia, weight loss, constipation, insomnia, AM-PM variations of mood, amenorrhea or impotency), extreme reduction of physical activity (may be mute or unresponsive), apathetic, no initiative, full of despair (feels everything is coming to an end), little insight, postural muscles seem to sag; delusions, illusions, and hallucinations are rare, but may occur.

- **Etiology** Loss, failure, guilt, low self-esteem, inability to handle anger (turns toward self, instead of outward to appropriate target). Pre-morbid personality usually contains a milder degree of feelings of low self-esteem than in psychotic depression, with a less harsh superego, less severe feelings of guilt and worthlessness, and more realistic perceptions.

Same as neurotic depression. Premorbid personality usually includes chronic low self-esteem, ambivalent feelings about self with harsh and punitive superego leading to feelings of guilt and depreciation of self, unrealistic perceptions of events, feelings. Closely linked with difficulty in interpersonal relations.

— **Reactive and endogenous depressions:**

Reactive (or exogenous)

Endogenous (aka physiological depression)

- **Precipitating event** Identifiable

Not evident or clearcut

- **Behaviors** Responds to environmental stimuli; weight loss less than 10 lbs; feels worse as day progresses; difficulty going to sleep; apathetic.

Does not respond to environmental stimuli; weight loss more than 10 lbs; feels worse in AM and better as day progresses; may sleep most of day; often awake at 4 or 5 AM; severely retarded thought and actions; responds to medications and ECT.

- **Etiology** Sudden onset, related to a loss

Onset 1–4 weeks, seems to come from nowhere; tends to be time-limited; possible biochemical aspect; person may have history of family members with depression.

- **Treatment:** since there is no right or wrong way to view or define depression, there is no single way to treat it. Somatic therapies of medications and/or ECT, plus some form of psychotherapy (short-term, crisis intervention, group or family therapy) are generally implemented. See NCPG #3:46, "Drugs: Psychotropic," and #3:47, "Drugs: Tranquilizers."
- **Nursing responsibilities** include assessing patient's symptom cluster, helping him to deal with painful feelings, assessing response to somatic therapies, providing support, and doing anticipatory planning to prevent and/or cope with future episodes.

Specific Considerations, Potential Patient Outcomes, and Nursing Actions:

1) Inability to Cope with Painful Feelings (e.g., Sadness, Grief, Guilt, Anger)

The patient will demonstrate increased ability to cope with painful feelings by accepting nurse's presence, sharing feelings with nurse and others, tolerating experiencing the feelings, exploring ways to cope with the feelings, tolerating reciprocal sharing of feelings with others, and resolving the feelings:

- build rapport & relationship with pt. by spending time with him at least twice daily; start with 5–10 minutes, & increase time as you & pt. can tolerate it; encourage pt. to identify & share feelings with you, accepting what s/he says; use silence; just the presence of a caring person is helpful when one is learning to cope with painful feelings; *avoid* reassurance;
- focus on pt.'s feelings; allow him to ventilate in ways that seem comfortable to him; share with pt. that the only way to get through the feelings is to stay with them & experience them;
- help pt. explore ways to cope with feelings; talk about alternate ways to express them, *e.g., to express anger:* try handball, racketball, hitting a punching bag or bed, shouting, singing, confronting with words, swearing, batacas, tearing up phone books, throwing sponges or bean bags; *to express guilt:* explore situation & persons with whom the pt. experiences guilt: "I feel guilty when I . . .," then have pt. try to replace the word "guilt" with "resentment;" explore feelings about this; most situations that involve guilt also involve feelings of anger & resentment; work on these feelings with pt.;
- explore with pt. the persons in his life with whom s/he is willing to share feelings; if there is no one, explore with him how this came about & his feelings about this situation; if s/he expresses dissatisfaction with having no one to share feelings with, explore ways to change situation; practice using role-playing or psychodrama to try alternative ways to initiate sharing of feelings;
- explore with pt. how s/he feels about listening to others' feelings; often people who have problems tolerating their own feelings tend to feel overwhelmed with others' feelings; practice sharing feelings of being overwhelmed & setting limits on listening to problems; if other pts. are willing & available, practice reciprocal sharing of feelings, with discussion of how to set limits & keep relationship;

— listen to pt.: focus on meaning of loss, somatic symptoms, feeling tone ("It seems like it just isn't worth it;" "You've had a hard time lately and you're learning to deal with your feelings;" "You've lost someone you loved and you're going through grief and mourning;" "Sounds like you remember the good parts and the rough parts of this relationship, & you're beginning to be ready to risk again.");
— give positive reinforcement to reality & realistic expectations.

2) Inability to Perform Self-Care Activities

The patient will resume self-care in grooming; will ingest adequate foods and fluids; will achieve adequate sleep-rest-activity pattern:
— assess activities of daily living & vegetative signs;
— identify problem areas & work out alternatives with pt. & health team; take care to consider individual preferences & needs; help pt. do things for self (many depressed pts. become dependent on others, but activity usually helps them to feel better);
— assess areas in which pt. is making own decisions & give positive reinforcement to self-enhancing ones; assist with decision-making when profoundly depressed; as depression lifts, expect pt. to make own decisions with support;
— weigh weekly (continued loss of weight may indicate deepening depression; weight gain may indicate decreased depression);
— work with pt. to plan activities of daily living in areas of:
   1) *personal appearance*: help pt. establish routine for bathing, care of hair, skin, nails, clothes; give positive reinforcement to any care of self;
   2) *food intake*: work with pt. to find acceptable eating pattern; if pt. is anorexic & apathetic to food, find out when this lessens; could you leave a thermos of hot chocolate, oatmeal cookies, crackers & cheese, 7-Up, etc., at bedside for small snacks at night or day?
   3) observe *sleeping habits*: help pt. establish a bedtime routine to promote rest & sleep; without enough sleep, exhaustion may occur & the mental state deteriorate; some depressed people seem to sleep continuously during the day & do not rest at night; work with pt. to mobilize self during day so will be able to rest at night;
   4) plan *work assignment with pt.* (daily responsibility for ward maintenance tasks helps to renew a sense of self-worth & purposefulness); simple tasks, such as emptying ashtrays, straightening chairs, putting away cards, games or crafts equipment with supervision may be appropriate for deeply depressed pts.; more difficult tasks can be gradually assigned as pt. tolerates;

5) assess *previous hobbies & pastimes* that pt. enjoyed (often depressed persons have few hobbies & haven't participated in recreational or crafts groups since schooldays); simple crafts that can be finished in one sitting give the pt. a therapeutic sense of accomplishment; group singing, poetry reading, painting, working with clay should be encouraged to assist pt. to become more comfortable in groups & to establish community & group socialization; pt. may need nurse's presence to tolerate group activities at first; simple exercises, walks, may progress to group sports;

6) assess *bowel habits* & work with pt. to choose roughage foods & sufficient fluids if constipated (often resumption of exercise & previous eating habits solves a constipation problem);

7) assess *pt.'s knowledge of AM-PM variations in mood* & depression; for pts. with endogenous depression, health teach that most pts. feel low in AM & better as the day progresses, especially if they mobilize themselves into activity; for pts. with reactive depression, health teach that their fatigue level affects their depression, so that as day progresses, they may become tired & feel more depressed; if so, they may need to rest in middle of day & do group work in AM, when they feel less depressed;

— if pt. is agitated, above nursing actions may help to rechannel his energy.

3) Self-Defeating/ Destructive Impulses (Related to Overwhelming Feelings of Low Self-Esteem, Hopelessness, & Helplessness)

The patient will demonstrate increased ability to control self-destructive behavior:

— assess pt.'s impulse control by restricting pt. to observable areas when first admitted; ask pt. if s/he has thought of hurting self or of suicide (see NCPG #3:38, "Suicide");

— remove potentially harmful items such as razor blades, scissors, meds, etc., on admission; sharp instruments can be used only with 1-to-1 supervision;

— establish a 1-to-1 relationship with pt.; assess potential for self-defeating acts; problem solve with pt. for alternative behaviors; use role-playing & psychodrama to practice new behaviors;

— work out plan for pt. to use when s/he feels that s/he is losing control of own impulses, e.g., contract with pt. that s/he will ask nurse to accompany him to exercise room so s/he can hit punching bag when angry at self or others; or contract to spend time with pt. when s/he experiences increased anxiety or depression, so that s/he can talk about feelings, cry, rage, & not be alone;

— give positive reinforcement by words & your presence when pt. follows through on contract to control impulses ("You really were aware that you were losing control and took good care of yourself by asking me to stay with you.");

	— retain hope & share it with pt. ("I know you are feeling low now; you're getting treatment and these feelings will lift.").
4) Social Relation- ships	The patient will strengthen ability to relate to others by increasing social interactions with staff and other patients:
	— assess interpersonal behaviors & help pt. define problem areas in social relationships, e.g., pt. who is hyper-critical of self & others can discuss & practice a softer, more accepting approach;
	— help pt. to look at situations where s/he may push people away out of fear of rejection (reject them before they reject him);
	— assess for feelings of powerlessness in everyday life situations; see NCPG #5:34, "The Patient Experiencing Powerlessness," for interventions;
	— practice social skills, use role-playing; give positive reinforcement.

Discharge Planning and Teaching Objectives/Outcomes

1) (Patient/Family/Significant Other) Can verbalize painful feelings s/he was experiencing on admission and can contrast them to those s/he is feeling now.
2) Has a realistic plan for self-care in activities of daily living, as well as for resuming usual job, home, or school roles.
3) Has a plan for follow-up care, e.g., doctor, nurse, mental health clinic, etc.
4) Has a written list of medications, schedule, and potential side effects; knows where and how to obtain refills and can state importance of taking medications as prescribed.

Recommended References

"Behavior Modification." *NCP Guide #5:37*, Nurseco, 1981.
"Communicating with Depressed Persons," by A. Swanson. *Perspectives in Psychiatric Care*, April/June, 1975:63–67.
"Coping with Lethargy," by R.D. Knowles. *American Journal of Nursing*, August 1981:1465.
"Depression: Adaptation to Disruption and Loss," by R. Drake & J. Price. *Perspectives in Psychiatric Care*, October/December 1975:163–169.
"Drugs: Psychotropic." *NCP Guide #3:46*, 2nd Ed., Nurseco, 1983.
"Drugs: Tranquilizers." *NCP Guide #3:47*, 2nd Ed., Nurseco, 1983.
"Handling Depression by Identifying Anger," by R.D. Knowles. *American Journal of Nursing*, May 1981:968.
"Intercepting the Depression Cycle . . . so Prevalent Among the Elderly," by P. Miller. *Geriatric Nursing*, July-August 1980:133–135.
"The Occurrence of Depression in Women and the Effect of the Women's Movement," by C.T. Beck. *Journal of Psychiatric Nursing*, November 1979:14–16.
"The Patient Experiencing Powerlessness." *NCP Guide #5:34*, Nurseco, 1981.
"The Patient with Manic-Depressive Psychosis." *NCP Guide #3:36*, 2nd Ed., Nurseco, 1983.
"The Patient who is Suicidal." *NCP Guide #3:46*, 2nd Ed., Nurseco, 1983.
"Responses to Loss: The Grief & Mourning Process." *NCP Guide #1:31*, 2nd Ed., Nurseco, 1980.

The Patient with Manic-Depressive Psychosis

Definition: Manic-depressive psychosis is an affective disorder characterized by recurring opposite emotional states of mania and depression.

LONG TERM GOAL: The patient will resume effective management of own life and will be able to identify those behaviors indicative of an approaching manic or depressive episode.

General Considerations:

— **Manifestations:** intense mood swings of elation or depression, lasting two to three months to two years, if untreated. The mood swings may be gradual or quite sudden.

— **Incidence and occurrence:** the reported sexual ratio is two females to one male; disorder may have a genetic predisposition. The first clear-cut episodes usually occur in the 30s, but careful history-taking often reveals that there were significant fluctuations in mood at an early age. Some patients seem to have an annual or seasonal pattern to their mood swings, while others follow a random course.

— The **manic-depressive syndrome** is considered to be an *endogenous depression*; recurrent attacks of mania with or without depression are called *bipolar depression*; recurrent attacks of depression with no manic attack are called *unipolar depression*.

— **Common behaviors** include:

- **manic phase:** an affect of euphoria and elation, impulsive behavior (e.g., sudden trips or spending money wildly), no worries, may neglect self; does not have time to eat, sleep, dress; increased verbal and motor activity. May have loose associations with "flight of ideas" (thought sequence characterized by rapid speech, disconnected change of topics; tends to be incomprehensible to listener);

- in **hypomania** (a milder form of mania), patient may eat voraciously, experience increased sexual interest, and go for long periods of time without sleep and without appearing fatigued;

- in a **fully-developed mania,** patient may experience delusions, unrealistic ideas of an expansive, grandiose nature; motor activity may increase to a degree that patient cannot focus on food, caring for self, or sexual performance; when this happens, the hyperactivity may become life-threatening since the patient does not eat, drink, or sleep; weight loss is common, speech is incoherent, activity is ceaseless and wild, and impulsive, destructive acts towards any person in the environment may occur;

- **depressive phase:** see "endogenous depression" in NCPG #3:35, "The Patient Experiencing Depression (Psychiatric)."

— **Prognosis** of an individual manic-depressive episode is good, even without treatment, provided that the patient does not suffer from complete physical exhaustion in the manic phase or commit suicide in the depressive phase. Manic-depressive illness is a self-limiting condition that may recur, as opposed to the chronic deterioration of schizophrenia.

— **Treatment** aim is to eliminate the extremes of the mood swings; lithium carbonate is frequently used for this purpose. Tranquilizers are given to control hyperactivity. Once the immediate psychotic state has improved, psychotherapy is utilized to enhance functioning and level of wellness. See NCPGs #3:46, "Drugs: Psychotropic," and #3:47, "Drugs: Tranquilizers."

— **Nursing responsibilities** include manipulating the environment to meet the patient's needs, working with patient to identify and resolve painful feelings, teaching patient/family/significant other regarding medications, and planning for discharge.

Specific Considerations, Potential Patient Outcomes, and Nursing Actions:

1) Hyper-activity, Verbal and Motor

The patient will demonstrate increased ability to control motor and verbal behavior:
— assess motor & verbal behaviors as unobtrusively as possible; set limits PRN;
— know that important cues for setting limits are: a care giver is worried about potential suicide, feels that pt. is saying, "please take over . . .;" or patient is upsetting self or others with own behavior;
— remove pt. from all stimulating, exciting, noisy, disturbing influences, while still providing ample space for him to move around; explain firmly & quietly that a staff member will stay with him while he paces, talks, etc.; engage in conversation with pt. as little possible; let him know that the therapeutic plan is to de-escalate the hyperactivity & to provide a quiet, safe place for him;
— assess if pt. is a danger to self or others: ask pt. specifically if s/he has any suicidal or homicidal thoughts; if "yes," report to MD, & ensure that pt. is staffed on a 1-to-1 basis (see NCPG #3:38, "The Patient who is Suicidal");
— be alert to pt.'s wish to leave hospital (most manic patients do not see the need for hospitalization or the danger to themselves); if pt. not on 1-to-1, have him stay in sight of staff;
— promote rest & sleep by limiting exciting influences, giving warm bath, back rub, etc.; give sedatives as ordered.

2) Loss of Interest in Self-Care

The patient will carry out own personal hygiene and grooming:
— see nursing actions for consideration #6, "Loss of Interest in Self-Care" in NCPG #3:37, "The Patient with Schizophrenia."

3) Associative Looseness

The patient will be able to communicate clearly with staff:
— see nursing actions for consideration #3, "Associative Looseness" in NCPG #3:37, "The Patient with Schizophrenia."

4) Unrealistic, Grandiose Ideas	The patient will express realistic ideas and plans:	

— do not talk to pt. about the grandiose ideas, since that is non-therapeutic & pt. may become more out of control; rather, provide limits with a quiet room, walking or talking quietly, keeping in mind that the pt. is experiencing feelings of being overwhelmed;

— look for the reality stimuli causing the stress & explore this with pt.; interpret reality by telling pt. you feel s/he must be very anxious right now; listen for any feeling tone in response & follow up on it.

5) Inability to Cope with Painful Feelings (Grief, Guilt, Sadness, Anger)

The patient will identify and talk about the painful feelings s/he is experiencing:

— know that pt.'s inability to cope with painful feelings comes to the foreground as manic behavior begins to lessen;

— see nursing actions for consideration #1, "Inability to Cope with Painful Feelings" in NCPG #3:35, "The Patient Experiencing Depression;"

— assess for feelings of powerlessness in everyday life situations; see NCPG #5:34, "The Patient Experiencing Powerlessness," for interventions.

6) Depressive Behaviors

Read NCPGs #3:35, "The Patient Experiencing Depression (Psychiatric)," and #3:38, "The Patient who is Suicidal."

Discharge Planning and Teaching Objectives/Outcomes

1) (Patient/Family/Significant Other) Can identify feelings and behaviors indicative of an approaching manic-depressive episode, and knows to contact doctor/clinic when this occurs.

2) Knows importance of expressing feelings to others in order to facilitate communications and understanding and to receive support during difficult times.

3) Can perform personal hygiene and grooming activities on a daily basis.

4) Can take own medicines, knows the purpose and potential side effects of each, and to call doctor/clinic if these occur. Has a supply of medicines, and knows how to obtain refills.

Recommended References

"Behavior Modification." *NCP Guide #5:37*, Nurseco, 1981.

"Drugs: Hypnotics & Sedatives." *NCP Guide #3:45*, 2nd Ed., Nurseco, 1982.

"Drugs: Psychotropic." *NCP Guide #3:46*, 2nd Ed., Nurseco, 1983.

"Drugs: Tranquilizers." *NCP Guide #3:47*, 2nd Ed., Nurseco, 1983.

"Handling Depression by Identifying Anger," by R.D. Knowles. *American Journal of Nursing*, May 1981:968.

"Lithium," by E. Harris. *American Journal of Nursing*, July 1981:1310–1315.

"Manic-Depression: An Overview," by D.L. Dixson. *Journal of Psychiatric Nursing*, June 1981:28–31.

"The Patient Experiencing Depression (Psychiatric)." *NCP Guide #3:35*, 2nd Ed., Nurseco 1983.

"The Patient Experiencing Powerlessness." *NCP Guide #5:34*, Nurseco, 1981.

"The Patient with Schizophrenia." *NCP Guide #3:37*, 2nd Ed., Nurseco, 1983.

"The Patient who is Suicidal (on a Psychiatric Unit)." *NCP Guide #3:38*, 2nd Ed., Nurseco 1983.

"Women and Mental Illness. A Sexist Trap?" by A. McGrory, *Journal of Psychiatric Nursing*, September 1980:13–19.

The Patient with Schizophrenia

Definition: Schizophrenia is a psychotic reaction manifested by fundamental disturbances in a person's interactions with people and ability to think and communicate clearly.

LONG TERM GOAL: The patient will regain some measure of independence in self-care, take own medicines, and demonstrate increased ability to communicate with others.

General Considerations

— **Incidence:** schizophrenia is a complex psychiatric problem, accounting for approximately one-half of the population in mental hospitals. Most persons with symptomatology of schizophrenia are able to maintain themselves in society and are never hospitalized.

— **Onset** occurs most frequently between the ages of 17 and 27. There are several theories of etiology and research in this area is continuing.

— **Acute vs. chronic:** the course of schizophrenia varies. Some patients have an acute break with reality; others begin with an acute stage, decrease symptoms while in the hospital, and then resume symptoms whenever stress increases. The latter course tends to become a chronic symptom pattern.

— **Types:**

1) *paranoid*—manifested by extreme suspiciousness and delusions; may feel that people are against him or that voices are threatening him or telling him to do dangerous or violent acts. Also may state that s/he believes s/he is Christ or some important figure.

2) *catatonic*—manifested by abnormal postural movements; in extreme cases, patient may become so inactive that s/he cannot move, take care of self or talk; this is called "catatonic stupor." At the other extreme, s/he may go into "catatonic excitement," manifested by excessive motor activity and extreme agitation; the patient does not eat or sleep and may become dehydrated and exhausted.

3) *simple*—manifested by total lack of any substantial relationships, lack of social skills, apathy; no overt delusions, hallucinations, or illusions.

4) *hebrephrenic*—manifested by inappropriate affect, giggling, unrelated smiling and laughter, regression to an earlier period of life. May have grandiose delusions and hallucinations. Often has disregard of social restrictions; may dress bizarrely, urinate and defecate at will, and masturbate in public.

5) *undifferentiated*—manifested by problems with reality testing, communications, thinking, and interpersonal relationships.

— **Symptoms** may vary widely according to the severity and type of schizophrenia. The classical four symptoms are: ambivalence, associative disturbance, autism, and affect impairment. Symptoms are usually broken into two categories: *cognitive* (e.g., disturbances of language and thought, distortion of body image, feelings of depersonalization, hallucinations, delusions) and *motor* (e.g., withdrawal and isolation from others, inefficiency in performance). As a result of this symptomatology, the person focuses his interest and attention mainly on self with resultant loss of social interaction, friendships, goal-oriented behavior. In severe disturbances, the patient becomes autistic and retreats into own world. The hospitalized schizophrenic is usually too disorganized and inefficient to maintain a job or school, to manage a home or own affairs.

— **Common behaviors** include:

1) *withdrawal*—people and events lose their meaning; the schizophrenic becomes indifferent to everything outside self, has no interest in other people or events; not in touch with reality enough to make goals.

2) *apathy with a flat (emotionless) affect*—emotions seem to be minimal or absent; feelings may be out of keeping with the event.

3) *associative looseness*—the schizophrenic's strange way of thinking and handling words makes it almost impossible for the observer to follow and understand what s/he is saying because the associations do not follow any logical sequence. This looseness with words is caused by autistic thinking; this thinking is so subjective and private that only the patient is aware of its meaning, and it is an extreme retreat into fantasy.

4) *ambivalence*—contradictory feelings of love, hate, fear that manifest in contradictory statements about a person or situation, or in the patient's inability to make decisions or express emotions. Ambivalence is a normal feeling that is greatly exaggerated in schizophrenic patients.

5) *impairment of process of reality testing*—as manifested by (a) *hallucinations*: an imaginary sense perception during which the patient sees, hears, smells, or tastes things in a distorted way; patient may report this or behavior may suggest imaginary perception. Behaviors in response to hallucinations include gestures, stereotyped mannerisms, actions that seem odd such as speaking to an empty room as if someone were present, nodding head, tilting head to one side; (b) *illusions*: misinterpretation of an actual sensory experience, manifested by patient's statement or behavior; (c) *delusions*: false, fixed belief that cannot be corrected by logic; manifested in dialogue, especially when the patient feels s/he is the subject of a conversation between others, and may be symbolic of feelings of guilt, insecurity, and alienation.

6) *loss of interest in personal grooming*—manifested by wearing same clothes daily, wearing oldest clothes, no makeup, lack of grooming for hair, nails, skin.
— **Treatment:** medication is the most effective type of treatment. With the advent of anti-psychotic drugs, many schizophrenic patients have been discharged from the hospital and are maintained in the community. Adherence to the prescribed medications is very important, as psychotic symptoms tend to reappear with a cutback in drugs; see NCPG #3:46 "Drugs: Psychotropic." Other forms of treatment include group, individual, occupational, recreational, and industrial therapy.
— **Nursing responsibilities** include interpreting and reinforcing reality to the patient, assisting patient to manage own life efficiently, supporting patient in setting up goals for self, and helping patient to achieve some level of independence.

Specific Considerations, Potential Patient Outcomes, and Nursing Actions:

1) Withdrawal The patient will learn to tolerate nurse's closeness and interest; will withdraw fewer times from contact with other persons:
— establish dialogue in order to be able to spend time, talk, & plan with pt.; demonstrate an accepting attitude;
— plan with pt. convenient times to spend together; include 1-to-1 as well as ward activities; listen & observe for non-verbal behaviors;
— use silence; share with pt. that you are willing to spend time without talking if s/he so chooses;
— observe pt.'s pattern of social interaction & attendance at ward activities;
— support pt. with words & with your presence during activities that s/he finds frightening or difficult;
— discuss with pt. alternate ways to spend the day; describe his behaviors in a non-threatening way & indicate that you realize his difficulties in coping with the milieu;
— as pt. improves, provide anticipatory guidance for discharge (e.g., if pt. is experiencing withdrawal from social situation, role play the situation); encourage pt. to explore & pursue social situations where s/he feels most comfortable.

2) Apathetic with Flat Affect The patient will share feelings with a staff or family member or another patient:
— observe pt.'s verbal & non-verbal expressions of feelings; share your observations in a non-judgmental way ("This is what I notice and I'm wondering what you're feeling right now?" or "You don't seem upset right now, but if someone spat at me, I'd be mad"—or other behavior of another pt.);
— explore pt.'s feelings with him, accepting his right to feel as s/he does, no matter how illogical the feelings seem to you;

— give positive reinforcement for any expression of feeling & stay with pt. during this time;

— work with pt. to explore new ways to express feeling, e.g., to express anger, try handball, racketball, hitting a punching bag or bed, shouting, singing, confronting with words, swearing, batacas, tearing up phone books, throwing sponges or bean bags;

— expect exaggeration of expression combined with uncomfortable feelings when practicing this new behavior or expressing feelings;

— plan with pt. alternate ways to use feelings both within hospital & after discharge;

— observe verbal & non-verbal behaviors that may indicate any interest in activities; give support to any expression of interest;

— work with family/significant other to continue facilitation of pt.'s expression of feelings after discharge.

3) Associative Looseness

The patient will learn to make his thinking understandable to others and initiate conversation with staff or other patients:

— listen to & chart patterns & symbols used in verbal communication; validate meaning with pt. before making an interpretation;

— look for patterns or themes in the pt.'s verbalization (e.g., "lovely princess in a tower;" "the dragons are trying to get me;" "I'm hooked up to all the TV stations and they control me . . .;"

— be aware that pt.'s conversation can be filled with both rational & psychotic statements out of sequence; define for the pt. those statements that are confusing to you, as a way to help keep him on the subject & facilitate communication & understanding;

— if pt. is having disassociated thoughts, talk about concrete realities, e.g., ward environment, eating, sleeping, & how s/he is feeling in the hospital;

— assign a permanent staff member to spend time each day interacting with & listening to the pt.; discuss goals & alternatives but avoid giving advice;

— discuss with pt. how his behavior affects & is viewed by others; point out, in a non-threatening way, how inappropriate behavior may alienate others.

4) Ambiva-
   lence

The patient will express and accept own ambivalent feelings:
— observe pt. for ambivalent feelings & attitudes; validate your observations ("Sometimes you hate your roommate & sometimes you love her; that's how you feel");
— discuss ambivalence as a normal state of being in all persons, that doesn't have to immobilize; accept pt.'s feelings of confusion or immobilization while continuing to work towards acceptance.

5) Impairment
   of Process
   of Reality
   Testing
   (Halluci-
   nations,
   Delusions,
   Ideas of
   Reference,
   Illusions)

The patient will learn to define and test reality; the patient will learn to control impulsive behavior dictated by hallucinations; the patient will dismiss the internal voices s/he hears:
— deal with & support reality: tell pt. your name, remind pt. where s/he is; be clear & concrete in your statements;
— listen carefully to pt.; tell him when you do & do not understand;
— respond to the pt.'s thought disturbance, keeping in mind that the pt. is experiencing feelings of being overwhelmed; look for the reality stimuli causing the stress (e.g., a visit from a family member might trigger a thought disturbance) and explore possibilities with pt.;
— look for & chart behaviors & environmental stimuli that precipitate and/or relate to pt. withdrawing into fantasy (when reality is too threatening, fantasy provides a comfortable retreat that will lower anxiety); accept pt.'s need for fantasy without supporting the context of it;
— when pt. is hallucinating, have him name the fact that s/he is anxious & connect the behavior with it;
— if pt. is experiencing hallucinations, illusions, delusions, or ideas of reference, interpret reality by telling him that you do not see or hear or believe these things, & that s/he must be feeling very anxious right now; do not talk to him about his delusions as that is non-therapeutic & pt. may become more out of control; rather, provide limits with a quiet room, walking or talking with pt., explore the basis for him feeling s/he is the subject of others' conversations, & explain the reality of the actual situation;
— observe pt. for behavior indicating s/he is hearing voices (e.g., nodding head or tilting it to own side, talking to people who are not present); when this occurs, ask pt. what is going on at this time (if you ask if s/he is hearing voices, s/he is apt to say "no"); if s/he is hearing voices, discuss what hearing voices does for him, i.e., takes him away from painful/frustrating reality of interchange & relationships with others ("Right now, you'd rather listen to the voices than talk with Mr.—, your wife, etc."); help pt. focus on things in the immediate environment; do not give status or recognition to the voices;

— ask pt. if s/he has control over the voices; if not, supply controls with 1-to-1 support, or meds (controls will make pt. feel more secure);

— know that pt. must dismiss the voices himself, and that s/he may be very anxious after this; when this occurs, alert staff so that all can provide extra support as temporary replacements for the voices.

6) Loss of Interest (in Taking Care of Self, in Personal Grooming, and in Self-Image)

The patient will maintain good personal hygiene; will learn to manage own life in terms of personal grooming, taking medications; will strengthen interpersonal relationships:

— ensure that pt. bathes or showers at least Q1–2 days, dresses each day, & that s/he keeps own clothes clean; have pt. use washer-dryer PRN;

— provide an opportunity for pt. to groom nails & hair, clean teeth; work with pt. to find an acceptable time & place for grooming activities; give positive reinforcement for good grooming & dress;

— observe & chart diet actually consumed; assess learning needs for balanced diet & teach PRN; use creative ways to encourage pt. to maintain adequate diet (juice, peanuts, milkshakes, cookie baking sessions, etc.):

— teach pt. the importance of taking meds daily; discuss their effect; as pt. improves, shift the responsibility of getting & taking meds to him, as preparation for discharge;

— observe physical condition & report problems to MD;

— plan with pt. ways s/he will maintain self after discharge (e.g., caring for clothing, transportation, food shopping & meal preparation, recreation & work/school); help him set personal goals & support him in these;

— provide daily outlets for productive activity, e.g., occupational or industrial therapy; give positive rewards for all efforts; ask pt. what s/he would like to achieve, & help with this goal;

— as discharge nears, discuss with pt. a follow-up care schedule, & develop a plan to use in case s/he feels depressed, out of touch with reality, spaced out, etc.;

— assess availability of significant others; include them in discharge planning if possible.

Discharge Planning and Teaching Objectives/Outcomes

1) (Patient/Family/Significant Other) Has a list and schedule of medications, can verbalize the importance of taking them as prescribed, knows potential side effects, and knows how to obtain refills.

2) Has an appointment for follow-up care with doctor/clinic/day-care center, etc.; knows to contact them if s/he feels a need before the appointment date. Can state behaviors of increased anxiety or withdrawal that should be reported to doctor.

3) Has a plan to maintain self on a daily basis that includes eating an adequate diet, maintaining personal grooming, and interacting with others.

4) Knows importance of expressing feelings to others in order to facilitate communication and understanding, and to receive support during difficult times.

5) Family/significant others are aware that patient often has difficulty expressing feelings, and have learned to work with him to facilitate understanding.

6) Knows community resources and support groups, e.g., half-way houses, rehabilitation and vocational training, day-care centers.

Recommended References

"Biochemical Aspects of Schizophrenia," by B. Stewart, *American Journal of Nursing*, December 1975:2176–2179.

"Drugs: Psychotropic." *NCP Guide #3:46*, 2nd Ed., Nurseco 1983.

I Never Promised You a Rose Garden, by H. Green. New York: Holt, Rinehart & Winston, 1964.

"The Miracle of Caring . . . A Mute Catatonic Schizophrenic," by A.B. Dormer. *Journal of Psychiatric Nursing*, August 1980:21–24.

"Working with Schizophrenic Patients." (A special section) *American Journal of Nursing*, June 1976:941–949.

The Patient who is Suicidal (on a Psychiatric Unit)

Definition: Suicide may be defined as an act to voluntarily end one's own life; it may be the ultimate act of self-hatred, or an attempt to control the time and circumstances of death. Suicide is a method of communication, a "cry for help," a visible sign that the person wishes to escape an intolerable situation and has run out of positive alternatives.

LONG TERM GOAL: The patient will be free of suicidal ideation, thoughts, and feelings, and will develop new alternatives to cope with the conditions that contributed to the suicidal state.

General Considerations:
— **Statistics:** suicide has ranked among the 12 leading causes of death in the US for several years; it is the third leading cause of death in the 15–19-year-old age group and the second leading cause of death on college campuses. Three times more males than females *commit* suicide; females *attempt* suicide more frequently than males.
— **Populations at risk:** suicide is higher in single, widowed, separated, and divorced people. In the US it is more prevalent in white than non-white persons; also high for migrants, foreign-born, the aged, and those living alone; is associated with alcoholism and homicide. Suicide in the aged is associated with physical and mental illness, social isolation, death of a loved one, loss of income or status (especially in retirement). Danger points for suicide are stressful situational or maturational events or passage through the usual developmental phases. Read NCPGs #2:31 & 2:35, "Crisis Intervention."
— **Common behaviors** include nagging lack of optimism and hope about the future, intense sense of unhappiness, depression, and inability to control own impulses; agitation and restlessness, which may increase as the person experiences loss of impulse control (loss of impulse control in some people may be accompanied by withdrawal, apathy, and immobility); helplessness and dependency; social isolation (few contacts with neighbors, family, or friends); intense loneliness (a subjective feeling unrelated to social isolation); marked hostility, anger, and powerlessness.
— **Warnings (or clues):** studies show that suicidal persons give many verbal and/or non-verbal warnings or clues of suicidal plans, e.g., giving things away that they usually need, making a will, checking on life insurance; pointed questions such as, "How do you go about giving your body to science? Does this hospital use kidneys or eyes donated before a person dies?" or statements concerning thoughts of death . . . "If I died, I'd want a white casket and white flowers," or even "Goodbye, nurse," which can be a significant statement if the timing or wording is different from usual. Statements such as, "I'm too far gone for anyone to help me," or, "The world's a jungle and I can't face it," give clues to the person's hopelessness and helplessness.

— **In assessing the risk** of a suicide attempt or of repeating a suicide attempt, a psychiatric diagnosis is one of the key prognostic factors. Frequently encountered diagnoses will be:

- *Depression*: patient may state "I deserve to be dead," . . . "My wife and children are better off without me," . . . "I just can't face it anymore." There is increased risk as an out-patient if (a) depressive symptoms are severe with marked change in ability to care for self or marked feelings of hopelessness or guilt; (b) patient is extremely agitated and impulsive; (c) is out of contact with reality; or (d) if there is a pattern of continuing suicidal ideation.
- *Schizophrenia*: high suicidal risk if patient is experiencing delusions or hallucinations; may include hostile voices that tell him to injure self.
- *Organic brain syndrome*: suicidal risk is increased if patient is repeating negative or self-defeating patterns, deals with stress by use of alcohol or drugs, demonstrates impulsive behavior, has limited adaptive responses, has mood swings, is confused, or if indicates s/he may have delusions, illusions, or hallucinations.
- *Personality disorders*: (1) hysterical personality—includes dependent behaviors and acting out; suicide often a gesture or power play. (2) Chronic alcoholic—demanding, dependent behavior with disordered interpersonal relationships; solves problems with alcohol, which increases vulnerability to negative and impulsive behaviors. (3) Antisocial personality—impulsive, demanding, and manipulative in egocentric way; has history of behavior harmful to others; suicide may be manipulation of social situation; patient may be threat to self and others.

— **Treatment** includes decreasing the overwhelming feelings of helplessness and hopelessness, increasing impulse control, and developing positive alternatives.

— **Nursing responsibilities** include prevention (by recognition of behaviors of persons at risk), assessment of lethality of intent, and working with patient/client to restore hope and develop positive alternatives. It also includes *providing self and other staff with a supportive environment,* since working with suicidal patients is emotionally draining and anxiety-producing. (This supportive environment includes daily supervision and informal discussion regarding feelings about suicide, death, hostility, anger, depression, and other painful emotions.) Developing an on-going relationship with a suicidal patient is an intense experience in which both persons in the relationship examine their existential feelings about the value of life and the meaning of life and death. It is an opportunity for the staff member to share her commitment to life, her hope and caring for the other person. If the staff member does not receive support and supervision, s/he will be unable to develop this kind of intense, caring relationship; both s/he and the patient will experience increased anxiety and will then have less energy to work toward hope and health.

Specific Considerations, Potential Patient Outcomes, and Nursing Actions:

1) Observation and Protection; Helpful Relationships

The patient will be safe from injury; will establish a trusting relationship and rapport with at least one staff member:

— assume responsibility for safety of pt. (*a priority*): inspect ward for potentially hazardous situations; make sure windows are shatterproof or use first floor facilities; remove sharp objects such as scissors, nail files, razor blades, & medication from pt.'s access (may be used only with 1-to-1 supervision);

— restrict pt. to observable areas of ward, deciding when s/he may leave unit with staff, visitors, or alone; use 1-to-1 staffing as needed;

— plan staffing so that unit is always covered by experienced staff, especially at staff meal times, breaks, vacations, change of shift; suicide occurs most often in hospital settings during change of shift, at mealtimes, or on weekends;

— assess for suicide plan & lethality: when, where, how, with what tools; plans are *more lethal* when they are specific: i.e., person has planned specific time and isolated place, or plans severe or self-mutilating act such as large amount of lethal meds; *less lethal* when plans are vague, or plans a minor dose of meds or superficial cut wrist in a place where can be discovered;

— assess intensity of wish to die & determination; pt.'s statements & affect are best indicators;

— assess past history: past unresolved losses, history of previous suicidal attempt in pt. or pt.'s family (previous attempt increases risk); is pt. in therapy & is therapist available? (pt. is at risk if therapist is on vacation or unavailable);

— assess pt.'s perception of situation & feelings about it & self; listen for pt.'s level of hope, view of situation as being intolerable, feelings of inadequacy in coping with present & past stresses, loss or expected loss, frustrations, feelings of unworthiness; *if pt. has attempted suicide*, listen for attitude about the attempt; is s/he sorry s/he didn't succeed & threatening to try again? does s/he regret the behavior & plan to come for help if s/he feels that s/he is going out of control?

— assess social network: does pt. have a significant other, e.g., close friend or family member? is this person available? is relationship under increased stress at this time or has there been a loss of this relationship? the more friends a person has, the stronger the support system;

— assess current life situation: ask pt. to describe it to you; look for stress situation, intensity of stress, losses, increased depression, loss of hope;

　　　　　　　　　— spend time with pt. to observe behaviors & begin building a trusting relationship; know that a relationship & rapport with staff is one of most important deterrents to suicide; know that this pt. has an intense need to trust, to be accepted, to increase self-esteem; respect, caring, & concern are vitally important to him.

2) Inability to Cope with Painful Feelings

The patient will identify and talk about painful feelings s/he is experiencing:
　　— see consideration #1, "Inability to Cope with Painful Feelings," in NCPG #3:35, "The Patient Experiencing Depression (Psychiatric)."

3) Inability to Perform Self-Care Activities

The patient will resume self-care in grooming; the patient will ingest adequate foods and fluids:
　　— if pt. suffers from insomnia, assign a staff person to check on him at ½-hour intervals & spend time with him during night; early morning hours may be most difficult time for this pt. & the time when s/he needs a nurse's presence the most;
　　— see consideration #2, "Inability to Perform Self-Care Activities," in NCPG #3:35, "The Patient Experiencing Depression (Psychiatric)," eliminating #7 of that section.

4) Intense Loneliness; Difficulty with Social Relationships

The patient will experience less loneliness; the patient will show increased ability to make contact in social relationships:
　　— see consideration #4, "Social Relationships," in NCPG #3:35, "The Patient Experiencing Depression (Psychiatric)."

Discharge Planning and Teaching Objectives/Outcomes
1) thru 4) Same as for "The Patient Experiencing Depression (Psychiatric)," NCPG #3:35.
5) (Family/Significant Other) Can identify high suicidal risk behaviors and has worked out a suitable crisis plan.

Recommended References
"Assessment of Suicidal Potential in Adolescents," by C.L. Tishler et al. *Journal of Emergency Nursing*, March/April 1980:24–26.
"Behavior Modification." *NCP Guide No. 5:37*, Nurseco, 1981.
"Crisis Intervention." *NCP Guide #2:35*, 2nd Ed., Nurseco, 1980.
"No Suicide Contract for Nurses," by B.G. Twiname. *Journal of Psychiatric Nursing*, July 1981:11–12.
"Nursing Care of a Suicidal Adolescent," by L. Wiley. *Nursing 80*, August 1980:64–66.
"The Patient Experiencing Depression (Psychiatric)." *NCP Guide #3:35*, 2nd Ed., Nurseco, 1983.
"The Patient Experiencing Powerlessness." *NCP Guide #5:34*, Nurseco, 1981.
"The Patient Needing Crisis Intervention." *NCP Guide #2:31*, 2nd Ed., Nurseco, 1980.
"Suicide: a Case for Investigation," by Sr. N. Loughlin. *Journal of Psychiatric Nursing*, February 1980:8–12.

The Patient who has Attempted Suicide
(and has been admitted to a Medical/Surgical Unit)

LONG TERM GOAL: The patient will recover from the suicidal attempt, and will establish a link to a mental health professional for continuing care.

General Considerations:
— Read NCPGs #3:38, "The Patient who is Suicidal (on a Psychiatric Unit)," and #3:35, "The Patient Experiencing Depression (Psychiatric)."
— **Incidence & occurrence:** 12.5 per 100,000 is about the world-wide and US average; approximately 200,000 attempts yearly in the US with 25,000 or more completed suicides (this figure may be nearly double since many suicides are reported as accidents.) Rates have increased over the past two decades. Twice as many men as women commit suicide, although women make more unsuccessful attempts. Rates for widowed and divorced persons are four to five times those of married couples. The singles rate is twice that of married, except the single female adolescent rate is lower than married female adolescent rate. Although still high, the suicide rate for elderly persons is decreasing somewhat, while increasing for adolescents—from four to twelve per 100,000 annually over the past 25 years. Protestants and non-religious people have higher rates than practicing Jews and Catholics. Rates are twice the national average for physicians, dentists, lawyers, business executives, and college students, especially if male, divorced, or in another high risk category. Rates are higher for whites compared to blacks, but urban black males are a higher risk group than formerly. Suicide is five times the national average in some Native American tribes.
— **Precipitating causes** of suicidal attempts form a chain of circumstances somewhat as follows:
1) a long standing history of problems or stressful events that escalate or a single critical event such as a real or threatened loss (of a loved one, job, prestige, money, health, hope, significant body part, etc.);
2) progressive failure of available adaptive techniques for coping, associated with reduced self-esteem;
3) progressive social isolation from meaningful affectionate relationships, associated with progressive unhappiness and growing depression; often there is a perceived lack of affection or acceptance from parents and/or peers accompanied by unbearable pain;
4) progressive hopelessness and despair; and
5) fantasies of death followed by internal justification of suicide to bridge the gap between self-destructive thoughts and concerted action. Sometimes this is viewed as emotional blackmail to punish significant others; sometimes this is a response to delusions of inner voices telling person to carry out act.

- **Attitudes of health care personnel** have a critical effect on the suicidal patient. Many general nursing unit care providers experience feelings of anger, frustration, unsympathetic attitudes, and fear of involvement while around patients who have attempted suicide. Since they are actively involved in life-preserving, life-prolonging measures, it is difficult to understand and accept patients who are trying to end theirs. Furthermore, attention-seeking behavior and special treatment demands of these patients tend to alienate staff. Rejection perceived by patient from staff only increases the patient's feelings of self-deprecation, worthlessness, helplessness, and hopelessness. Changes in the patient's attitude toward self and the feeling of hope come primarily via therapeutic staff-patient relationships. It is therefore incumbent upon health care providers to recognize their negative feelings, to share them with each other, and to receive counseling and encouragement from colleagues so that an empathic understanding and a positive therapeutic attitude may prevail.
- **Essential skills** of interviewing, counseling, and utilizing crisis intervention philosophy and methods need to be practiced by the general nursing staff caring for the suicidal patient. Refer to NCPGs #2:35, "Crisis Intervention," and #1:31, "Responses to Loss: the Grief and Mourning Process."
- **Suicides occur in hospitals** at a much greater rate than in the general community: three and a half times higher for medical and surgical patients and 30 times higher for neuro-psychiatric patients. Jumping or hanging are the most frequently used methods. Legal implications necessitate clearly written hospital policies and guidelines for safeguarding suicidal patients. These policies should cover areas of lethality assessment, environmental precautions, safe care procedures, staff communications, attitudes and behavior, and record documentation. Courts now recognize "therapeutic risk" to achieve therapeutic goals, so standards of practice and care need not be rigid or repressive. Rather, guidelines should provide staff with competent, community-based professional practices that, when followed, help a staff feel secure, confident, and guilt-free, regardless of patient outcome.
- **Treatment aims** to save life and restore bio/psycho/social stability; to promote feelings of self-worth and hope; and to refer patient appropriately and promptly for psychotherapy.
- **Nursing responsibilities** include carrying out life-saving measures to restore physiological homeostasis; providing a safe, protective, supportive environment to prevent another suicide attempt; establishing a warm, caring, nonjudgmental relationship in which contact and communication are consistently and continuously maintained; assessing suicide potential including lethality of plan and risk factors; supporting and counseling family and friends; initiating a therapeutic plan in partnership with patient, family or friends, physician, and mental health consultants; documenting for legal reasons that suicidal behavior is recognized, lethality assessment is made, precautionary safety measures have been taken, consultation has been obtained, and all medical orders and hospital guidelines for suicide prevention have been followed; and making appropriate referrals to community resources PRN.

Specific Considerations, Potential Patient Outcomes, and Nursing Actions:

1) Restoration of Physiological Homeostasis

The patient will stabilize physiologically, free of preventable complications; the patient will recover from the suicide attempt in a safe, nonjudgmental environment:

— assist with resuscitation measures, gastric lavage, ECG monitoring, etc., as the pt.'s condition indicates;

— maintain pt.'s life by measures dictated by state of consciousness & condition: e.g., administer O_2, keep airway patent with PRN suctioning, have pt. cough, deep breathe, turn from side to side at least Q1H;

— if pt. comatose, maintain Foley catheter, body alignment, & skin integrity with usual nursing measures; monitor level of consciousness & corneal reflexes; perform neuro checks at least Q1H;

— establish & maintain patent IV line; record I&O; chart urine output Q1H;

— monitor cardiac function & vital signs on a continuous basis, reporting significant changes promptly to MD;

— if pt. has poisoned or overdosed self, determine, if possible, type & amount of drug taken as well as its expected side effects; it is important to note not only if it was a lethal dose but whether the pt. *thought* it was a lethal dose; assist with appropriate medical treatment & prescribed medication administration;

— do not be too busy carrying out life-saving functions to arrange to give (or someone else to give) emotional support to victim, family, & friends; know that some emergency centers have a clinical nurse specialist on call or access to 24-hour staff at nearby mental health centers; know that such immediate psychiatric first aid can mean the difference between recovery & another attempt or completed suicide.

2) Painful Feelings

The patient will identify and reveal the painful feelings s/he is experiencing; the patient will verbalize perception of own current situation and how it happened; the patient will express a lessening of anxiety, helplessness, hopelessness, and worthlessness:

— listen to what pt. says, allowing uninterrupted talk or long silences without challenging statements, without giving advice, without chastising; do not support denial or unreality, but rather share how you see it (e.g., "This is what I hear you saying and this is what I think is happening or how I see it."); do not probe into unconscious motivation, leave this for psychotherapeutically trained specialist; be nonjudgmental, nondirective in approach; promise confidentiality;

— do not sidestep issue of suicidal attempt; recognize the seriousness of the unbearable pain pt. is obviously experiencing; do not be afraid to discuss pt.'s suicidal behavior & thoughts; acknowledge that s/he is a troubled, unhappy person; express your willingness and availability to listen because you care (e.g., "I am concerned about you!", "I want to help," "Things must look pretty hopeless to you right now.");

— establish, if possible, a relationship with pt. that expresses warmth, sensitivity, honesty, & concern in a consistent, continuing manner;

— assess pt.'s attitude re: failure of suicide attempt & the nature of the attempt ("What did you think would happen when you . . .?"); evaluate lethality & the immediate risk of another attempt;

— distinguish between rational pts.' communication with you & those who have lost touch with reality; know that those pts. having visual or auditory hallucinations, delusions, or agitated depression are especially vulnerable to self-destruction; observe very closely & do not leave unattended even when pt. is using bathroom or having diagnostic tests; as soon as possible, arrange for transfer of pt. to a psychiatric unit or facility;

— assume responsibility for pt.'s safety; follow hospital procedures for suicide precautions & ascertain that all persons coming in contact with pt. clearly understand restrictions; teach staff to be particularly alert when medications are given (the medication carts & trays are never unattended); take special care during changes of shift or other busy times when staff may be preoccupied with an emergency; know hospital policy re: 1-to-1 staffing or permission for family/friends to be in attendance; assure pt. s/he is safe from own self-destructive impulses; know that pts. usually take these safety precautions well because they view them as an indication that staff really cares about them & takes their suicidal threats seriously;

— rally the support of caring family members &/or friends; allow them to ventilate own feelings re: suicide & the pt., so that they can work more effectively with pt.; provide support & encouragement PRN;

— assess nursing staff's feelings & attitudes toward pt., as well as your own; arrange PRN pt. care conferences with psychiatric clinical specialist to promote therapeutic staff-pt. relationships.

3) Patient/ Family Education & Discharge Planning

The patient expresses willingness to participate in professional mental health counseling and follow-up for at least six months or as long as needed:

— discuss discharge plans with pt.; does s/he accept need for mental health counseling? point out that such follow-up will strengthen own coping strategies & independence;

— ask pt. what s/he is willing to do to help self; will s/he talk on a regular basis with a school counselor, teacher, clergyperson, social worker, marriage & family counselor, mental health specialist, psychologist or psychiatrist? know that it is important to find a referral that is acceptable to pt. & arrange for a back-up resource in case of urgent need; after consultation with physician, family, friends, initiate appropriate referrals & arrange first contact before the pt. leaves hospital;

— know that a directory listing of all suicide prevention & crisis intervention centers throughout country is available from American Association of Suicidology, 220 West 20th Ave., San Mateo, CA 94403; arrange for obtaining one for your own or nursing staff's usage.

Discharge Planning and Teaching Objectives/Outcomes

1) (Patient/Family/Significant Other) Has the telephone numbers of the nearest Suicide Prevention or Crisis Intervention Center, Hot Line, Help Line, and therapist.

2) Has a specific appointment time and place for follow-up mental health counseling therapy (required by law for at least three months in some states).

3) (Family/Significant Other) Is aware of the clues or danger signals of suicidal urges (refer back to "General Considerations") and indicates that s/he will seek immediate professional help and stay with person until help has been obtained.

Recommended References

"Adolescent Suicide," by M. Allison and T. Linson. *Journal of Nursing Care*, September 1981:7–9.

"Cancer and Suicide," by M. Maxwell. *Cancer Nursing*, February 1980:33–38.

"Crisis Intervention: Adaptation to General Nursing." *NCP Guide #2:35*, 2nd Ed., Nurseco, 1980.

"Deliberate Self-Poisoning in Children and Adolescents," by R. Tyrrell. *Issues In Comprehensive Pediatric Nursing*, June 1980:45–54.

"Emergency Psychiatry: An Update," by A. Slaby. *Hospital and Community Psychiatry*, October 1981:692–693.

"Helping Suicidal Adolescents," by R. Leon. *Consultant*, September 1980:115, 118, 119.

"Nursing Care of a Suicidal Adolescent," by C. Welz-Ritchie et al. *Nursing 80*, April 1980:56–59.

"Pathological Identification as a Cause of Suicide on an Inpatient Unit," by M. Sacks and S. Eth. *Hospital and Community Psychiatry*, January 1981:36–43.

"The Patient Experiencing Depression (Psychiatric)." *NCP Guide #3:35*, 2nd Ed., 1983.

"The Patient Needing Crisis Intervention." *NCP Guide #2:31*, 2nd Ed., Nurseco, 1980.

"The Patient who is Suicidal (on a Psychiatric Unit)." *NCP Guide #3:38*, 2nd Ed., Nurseco, 1983.

"Responses to Loss: the Grief and Mourning Process." *NCP Guide #1:31*, 2nd Ed., Nurseco, 1980.

"Spotting and Stopping the Suicide Patient," by R. Reubin. *Nursing 79*, April 1979:83–85.

"The Suicidal Adolescent," by N. Hart and G. Keidel. *American Journal of Nursing*, January 1979:80–83.

"Suicide: A Case For Investigation," by Sister N. Loughlin. *Journal of Psychiatric and Mental Health Services*, February 1980:8–12.

"Suicide by Accident." *Emergency Medicine*, April 15, 1981:128–130.

"Suicide Prevention in the Hospital," by N.L. Farberow. *Hospital and Community Psychiatry*, February 1981:99–104.

"Suicide: The Ultimate Cry for Help," by C. Law; Part 2 "How Nurses Can Answer," by C. Reguero. *The Journal of Practical Nursing*, January 1979:18–22.

Acid-Base Balance

General Considerations:
— As with fluids and electrolytes, an **acid-base imbalance** is common to many patients in the health system. It is usually secondary to another condition or illness and often takes priority in treatment since acid-base balance is of utmost importance in maintaining the proper environment for cellular function and survival.
— **Acid-base** refers to the acidity or alkalinity of extracellular fluid (ECF). An *acid* is a substance that *donates* or gives up hydrogen ions. Acids normally generated by metabolism are of two types:
   1) *Volatile*: carbonic H_2CO_3 (the result of oxidation of glucose) dissociates into H_2O and CO_2. The CO_2 can be rapidly excreted by the lungs.
   2) *Fixed*: consist mostly of phosphates and sulphates (as a result of protein metabolism). The hydrogen ions must be buffered and excreted by the kidneys.
   A *base* is a substance that *accepts* hydrogen ions.
— **pH is a measure of hydrogen ion (H$^+$) concentration** of a solution and reflects the *acidity or alkalinity of the solution*. A chemically neutral solution is 7.0; an acidic one is 1.0 to 7.0; alkaline is 7.0 to 14.0. Normal blood pH is 7.35 to 7.45 (slightly alkaline). A pH below 7.35 indicates acidosis or an excess of H$^+$ ions. A pH above 7.45 indicates alkalosis or a deficit of H$^+$ ions. The principal determinant of acid-base balance is the ratio of bicarbonate (HCO_3) to carbonic acid (H_2CO_3):

$$pH \text{ (units)} = \frac{HCO_3 \text{ mEq/L}}{H_2CO_3 \text{ mEq/L}} = \frac{24}{1.2} = \text{ratio of } \frac{20}{1}$$

— **As acids or bases are formed** by metabolism or administered, the body must first protect its acid-base status against the effects of their accumulation and then dispose of them from the body by excretion or metabolism. A *buffer* or base bicarbonate is a complex formed when sodium, potassium, calcium, or magnesium combines with bicarbonate, e.g., $NaHCO_3$. *A buffer binds or releases H$^+$ ions and minimizes deviations of pH.*
— **Maintenance of acid-base balance** is controlled by three regulatory systems: (1) chemical buffers, (2) lungs, and (3) kidneys. When an imbalance occurs, the body attempts to correct it with these systems.
   • **Chemical buffers:** (1) *ECF buffers* are the fastest acting and provide immediate protection *within fractions of a second* to compensate against changes in H$^+$ ion in the ECF. The major buffers are the bicarbonate system (the 20:1 ratio of HCO_3 to H_2CO_3), hemoglobin, and plasma proteins. (2) *Intracellular* (ICF) buffers act more slowly, *2 to 6 hours*, and utilize ICF proteins and phosphates as the major buffers.

- **The lungs** attempt to regain acid-base balance by changing the rate and depth of respirations. If the body is too alkaline, the lungs will reduce respirations to retain CO_2 ($CO_2 + H_2O \rightarrow H_2CO_3$); if too acid, respirations will increase to blow off CO_2 ($H_2CO_3 \rightarrow CO_2 + H_2O$). This regulatory system is operative *within several minutes*.
- **The kidneys** provide the most thorough control of acid-base balance, and the ultimate restoration of chemical buffers are dependent upon them. They act by selective regulation of HCO_3 and H^+ in three ways: by retaining bicarbonate (HCO_3) otherwise lost in the urine; by the buffering of hydrogen ions by urinary phosphate (NaH_2PO4) resulting in the loss of H^+ from the body into the urine; and by the trapping of H^+ by urinary ammonia for excretion as ammonium (NH_4) in the urine. The result is urine with an H^+ concentration 1000 times greater than blood and a pH of about 6.0. Kidney regulation of acid-base balance starts rapidly but may *take hours to days to complete*.

— **Arterial Blood Gas Studies**

- The overall acid-base status (pH) of blood is determined by measuring arterial blood, which (after leaving the lung) reflects the status of lung function with regard to CO_2 as well as "metabolic" status.
- Arterial blood must be collected anaerobically, and determinations must be made at body temperature since pH and pCO_2 are affected by air and temperature.
- Prepare the patient carefully for this procedure; anxiety may result in hyperventilation that will alter the blood gas concentration.
- Blood is drawn from an indwelling catheter in the brachial, radial, femoral, or temporal artery. If an indwelling catheter is not in place, a femoral punch is required. Nurses oftentimes may draw arterial samples from an indwelling catheter, but not when a punch is required.
- Most laboratories require 2 to 2.5 ml of unclotted blood for arterial gas studies. A plastic cap must be placed over the syringe immediately after collection to prevent air from entering the syringe; it is then brought immediately to the laboratory.
- Note on the requisition slip if patient is receiving O_2 therapy; state rate and route of administration.
- *Normal blood gas values* (lab values may vary slightly between institutions):

pH	7.35– 7.45	HCO_3	22.00–26.00 mEq/L
pCO_2	35.00–45.00 mmHg	H_2CO_3	1.02– 1.38 mEq/L
pO_2	varies with pH—about 90 mmHg		

— **Nursing responsibilities** include being knowledgeable of the acid-base concept, being alert to signs and symptoms of an imbalance and reporting them to the physician, and initiating appropriate nursing actions.

— **Major imbalances** occur when the body's regulatory systems are ineffective, and external intervention is required. *Seen in their early uncompensated phase*, these are:

	Respiratory Component (plasma pCO$_2$)	Metabolic Component (plasma HCO$_3$)	Blood pH
Metabolic Acidosis	Normal	Decreased	Decreased
Metabolic Alkalosis	Normal	Increased	Increased
Respiratory Acidosis	Increased	Normal	Decreased
Respiratory Alkalosis	Decreased	Normal	Increased

Metabolic Acidosis

Defect

The retention of fixed acids in the ECF or the loss of bicarbonate (base).

Common Causes

Any clinical event that results in (a) an *acid excess* (e.g., diabetic acidosis, uremia, lactic acidosis in shock) or (b) *loss of base* (e.g., diarrhea, infection, inadequate caloric intake). Precipitating conditions: shock, liver disease, advanced circulatory failure, salicylate overdose, acute renal failure, dehydration, intestinal or biliary obstruction, hyperthyroidism; frequently complicated by hyperkalemia (as H$^+$ accumulates and diffuses through cells and body fluids, K$^+$ moves out of cells to maintain intracellular electrical neutrality). The compensatory mechanism involves the respiratory elimination of CO$_2$ (Kussmaul respirations) and the renal retention of bicarbonate.

Signs & Symptoms

Depression of CNS, headache, lethargy, anorexia, N&V, diarrhea, drowsiness, twitching, convulsions, hyperventilation, stupor, Kussmaul-type breathing, semi-consciousness

Lab Findings

- plasma pH *below* 7.35
- urine pH *below* 6.0

Metabolic Alkalosis

An excessive loss of hydrogen ion or an excess intake or retention of bicarbonate ion.

Any clinical event that results in *excessive intake of bicarbonate* (e.g., excess alkali ingestion in patients with ulcer disease); (b) *loss of fixed acid*, (e.g., prolonged emesis or NG suction, gastric lavage); or (c) *decrease in extracellular K* due to use of thiazide diuretics or hyperaldosteronism. The compensatory mechanisms include renal bicarbonate excretion, suppression of ammonia formation, and retention of hydrogen ion. Minimal respiratory compensation with CO$_2$ retention. This is the only acid-base disturbance where the basic defect and the compensatory mechanism involve the same system, i.e., the kidneys.

Overexcitability of CNS, N&V, diarrhea, confusion, irritability, agitation, possible coma & convulsions; others may be restlessness, muscle twitching.

- plasma pH *above* 7.45
- urine pH of 7.0

Metabolic Acidosis
- plasma bicarbonate *below* 25 mEq/L (adults)
- plasma bicarbonate *below* 20 mEq/L (children)
- serum CO_2 *below* 22 mmEq/L
- pCO_2 *below* 40 mmHg if compensating
- serum K often elevated
- pO_2 normal

Treatment Measures

To eliminate causative factor(s), an IV of Na bicarbonate may be given to increase the buffer base of the blood. In renal failure, peritoneal or hemodialysis may be used.

Nursing Responsibilities

- Keep Na bicarbonate, insulin, and IV 50% glucose ready for emergency use.
- Institute safety precautions for convulsions and coma.
- Maintain an accurate I&O record.
- Observe for changes in skin, vital signs, eye balls (sunken or protruding); monitor frequently.
- Check serum K level (due to H^+/K^+ shift, it may be elevated during early compensatory stages and it may drop as acidosis is corrected); observe for signs of hyperkalemia (hyperreflexia, twitching, bradycardia, ventricular fibrillation) and/or hypokalemia (diminished reflexes, weak pulse, falling BP, SOB, shallow respirations, vomiting).
- Do preventive health teaching; in diabetes, stress importance of adhering to diet and drug regimes.
- Be aware of changes in arterial blood gas status.

Metabolic Alkalosis
- plasma bicarbonate *above* 29 mEq/L (children)
- plasma bicarbonate *above* 25 mEq/L (adults)
- serum CO_2 *above* 32 mEq/L
- pCO_2 *above* 40 mmHg if compensating
- decreased serum K and Cl
- pO_2 normal

Aimed at correcting the pH imbalance and eliminating the underlying cause(s). Measures include: replacement of K & Cl orally or IV; medicines to promote excretion of excess bicarbonate in the kidneys; ingestion of acidifying solutions (e.g., ammonium chloride) to increase available acids in the serum.

- Institute safety precautions for coma and convulsions.
- Maintain accurate I&O record.
- Monitor vital signs.
- Know and observe for signs of *hypokalemia*.
- Do preventive health teaching, especially to high-risk patients (e.g., those taking soda water for ulcers or gastric acidity, patients with CHF taking diuretics).
- Be aware of changes in arterial blood gas status.

	Respiratory Acidosis	**Respiratory Alkalosis**
Defect	Alveolar hypoventilation with resultant retention of CO_2 (decrease in amount of CO_2 expired by the lungs).	The elimination of carbon dioxide as a result of alveolar over-ventilation (increase in amount of CO_2 expired by lungs).
Common Causes	(a) *Perfusion defects* (chronic pulmonary CHF with pulmonary congestion, disease e.g., emphysema, asthma, bronchiectasis; acute pulmonary disease e.g., pneumonia, severe pulmonary edema, atelectasis, an obstructing foreign body); (b) *depression of respiratory center* due to drugs, trauma. The compensatory mechanism is renal by the retention of bicarbonate, excretion of hydrogen ion and ammonia, since the defect is respiratory.	Sepsis, central nervous system diseases, overventilation with mechanical ventilators, pain, hysteria, lack of O_2. The compensatory mechanisms include renal excretion of bicarbonate, suppression of ammonia formation, and retention of hydrogen ions.
Signs & Symptoms	Decreased ventilation, disorientation, somnolence, changes in sensorium, weakness, coma; with increased hypoxia, the patient develops diaphoresis, restlessness, rapid irregular pulse. Cyanosis is an advanced sign.	Rapid, deep respirations; patient often has high anxiety and fear.
Lab Findings	<ul><li>plasma pH *below* 7.35</li><li>urine pH *below* 6.0</li><li>pCO_2 *above* 40 mmHg</li><li>elevated serum K</li><li>pO_2 normal or low</li><li>plasma bicarbonate above 27 mEq/L if compensating</li></ul>	<ul><li>plasma pH *above* 7.45</li><li>urine pH *above* 7.0</li><li>pCO_2 *below* 40 mmHg</li><li>decreased serum K</li><li>pO_2 usually normal</li></ul>
Treatment Measures	Establishment of adequate airway; assisted ventilation to increase aeration of the lungs (e.g., IPPB); control of	Elimination of inciting cause, reassurance, sedation; in severe cases, controlled ventilation with a volume-

Respiratory Acidosis

secretions (e.g., postural drainage); and avoidance of sedation.

Respiratory Alkalosis

cycled respirator. *Oversedation must be avoided* because sudden respiratory depression could lead to hypoventilation, acute respiratory acidosis, hypoxemia, and cardiac arrest.

Nursing Responsibilities

- Reduce restlessness by improving ventilation rather than by giving medicines; avoid giving sedatives, hypnotics, or tranquilizers as they reduce respirations.
- Help patient to turn, cough, and deep breathe (or use blow bottles) frequently.
- Suction PRN to maintain a patent airway.
- Increase oral fluids (check with MD for amount) in order to liquefy secretions.
- Monitor vital signs; be aware that an increased pulse rate may mean increasing acidosis.
- Observe for signs of increasing respiratory distress and report any to MD.
- Be aware of changes in arterial blood gas status.

- Stay with patient until breathing eases and acute anxiety subsides somewhat.
- Give medicine as ordered and observe for response.
- Observe for signs and symptoms of other conditions that may be masked by respiratory alkalosis.
- Be aware of changes in arterial blood gas status.

Recommended References

"The ABC's of ABG's or How to Interpret a Blood Gas Value," by K. Shrake. *Nursing 79*, September 1979:26–33.
"Acute Respiratory Insufficiency," by H. Sweetwood. *Nursing 77*, December 1977:24–31.
Fluids & Electrolytes: A Practical Approach, 2nd Ed., by C.V. Strout, C. Lee, & C. Schaper. Philadelphia: Davis, 1977.
Fluids & Electrolytes with Clinical Applications, 2nd Ed., by J. Kee. New York: Wiley, 1978.
"Interpreting Arterial Blood Gases," by L. Nielsen. *American Journal of Nursing*, December 1980:2197–2201.
"Metabolic Acid-Base Disorders, a Programmed Instruction Unit. Part I: Chemistry & Physiology," by S. Cohen. *American Journal of Nursing*, October 1977:1–32. "Part II: Physiological Abnormalities and Nursing Actions." *American Journal of Nursing*, January 1978:1–20. "Part III: Clinical and Laboratory Findings." *American Journal of Nursing*, March 1978:1–16.
"A Quick Review on Using Blood-Gas Determinations," by D.J. del Bueno. *RN*, March 1978:68–70.
"Symposium on Fluid, Electrolyte, and Acid-Base Balance." *Nursing Clinics of North America*, September 1980:535–646.

Back Care

LONG TERM GOAL: The patient will improve posture and use proper body mechanics when standing, walking, sitting, lying, lifting, working or playing; s/he will be able to prevent or minimize recurrence of low back pain due to injury.

General Considerations:

— Conscientiously practice suggestions and recommended positions given below until they become part of your natural automatic body functioning.

— Do not begin work or sports activities without a brief "warm-up" period, which should include a warm bath or shower and several stretching exercises.

— Be aware of your back. Avoid sudden or twisting movements.

— Learn to avoid and control muscular strain caused by fatigue, emotional tension, or quick chilling of a perspiring body. Wear protective clothing. Try to avoid overexertion and stressful situations. Explore methods of relaxation that are feasible and useful for you.

— Change positions every hour or as necessary to maintain adequate circulation and oxygenation of tissues. Take regular short walks (few minutes) during long hours of driving, sitting, or standing in one place.

— Plan for small amounts of regular exercise, sports activities, or work. Avoid weekend excesses.

— Do back care exercises (see NCPG #3:42) at least once, preferably twice, daily. Walk or swim at least 15–20 minutes at least three times weekly (daily when possible).

— Know that habitual wearing of skin-tight jeans, girdles, or back and abdominal supports will cause weakening of abdominal muscles. If these are necessary in your life, compensate with regular muscle-strengthening exercises on a daily basis.

— Do not do yard work, snow shoveling, or vacuuming when your back is "acting up" or when you are tense, tired, hurried, or angry.

— Control overweight. Obesity is a common cause of back aches.

Specific Suggestions:
— **Standing**
  - Practice maintaining a correct standing position: feet slightly apart facing straight ahead, weight balanced evenly on both feet, legs and knees straight but not tensed, abdomen pulled in, hips tucked under, small of back flattened as if pressing it into a wall, chest raised, shoulders back but not hyperextended, head up with neck straight and chin in, but not down.
  - Avoid standing for more than 30 minutes whenever possible. Use a foot stool to raise one foot for short periods to relieve swayback strain.

— **Walking**
  - Wear low-heeled shoes as much as possible; avoid habitual use of high-heeled shoes as they tilt pelvis and throw it out of line.
  - Walk in an even, rhythmic stride that is comfortable for you; swing arms freely and naturally; avoid carrying one-sided loads (such as heavy tote bags, children, or camera gear), using front or back pack bags to distribute load evenly. Breathe deeply while walking, holding chest up, abdomen in, head up, shoulders back, and chin in. Do not lean into walk or hunch forward.

— **Sitting and Driving**
  - Sit with back against straight (or nearly straight) back chair or seat. Move chair close to work to avoid leaning forward.
  - Avoid sitting in deep-cushioned sofas or armchairs; avoid swivel chairs, chairs on rollers, chairs too high or too low for proper sitting posture, and chairs with backs at greater than 100° slant.
  - Keep feet flat on floor or slightly crossed at ankles only, for occasional periods. Chair should be low enough that feet touch floor without reaching and that knees are slightly higher than hips, in order to flatten back and to prevent swayback strain. Footstools should be used when chair height cannot be readily adjusted. Avoid keeping legs straight out on an ottoman. Do not cross legs above the knees.
  - Do not carry a bulging wallet in back pocket as it throws posture off, causes pressure on the sciatic nerve, and may produce pain down the leg.
  - When driving, keep the seat sufficiently forward so that spine remains vertical and straight. Avoid sitting lop-sided, with one arm on the window edge. Keep both hands on the wheel. Do not slump or lean forward to drive. Use belts, shoulder harness and headrest to protect from sudden jolts and injuries as well as to prevent slouching. Stop every hour or so to walk around.
  - When getting in and out of car, swing legs as a unit. Avoid twisting back.

— **Lying (Resting and Sleeping)**
  - Use a firm mattress and a bedboard or box springs. Avoid lying on sofas, sofa-beds, cots, or hammocks (sleeping on a floor is preferable to these unsupported beds).
  - Do not lie on your stomach as it increases swayback strain and pain.
  - Lie on side with both knees bent or on back with legs elevated. Elevate legs in a bent-knee position with pillows, cushions, or folded blankets to keep back flattened against mattress. Elevate head and shoulders on a low, soft pillow.
  - When getting out of bed, turn to side with knees bent; push with hands to a sitting position while swinging legs over edge of bed.

— **Lifting and Working**
  - Be sure that path and floor are clear of hazards and feet are secure.
  - Always get help for loads that are more than one-third of your weight.
  - Push, rather than pull, large or bulky objects; roll or slide them when possible. Use luggage carts, dollies, mechanical patient lifts and other backsaving measures whenever possible.
  - Squat to stoop, bending hips and knees; never bend over at waist with straight legs. Do not turn slightly to one side to reach, put down, or pick up anything; always face object directly. Balance object's weight evenly in both arms. Hold close to body. Stand slowly. When possible, try to avoid lifting objects above your shoulder level (or heavy objects above waist level).
  - Use step ladders for reaching over head. Keep buttocks tucked under and refrain from arching back as you reach. Always try to keep back just barely rounded.
  - Kneel to work near floor. When using tools, keep them close to the body. Avoid long reaches with pulls, twists of the body, leaning to back or side, and jerky movements of torso. Always face your work and turn by pivoting your feet first.

Recommended References
"Back Exercises." *NCP Guide #3:42*, 2nd Ed., Nurseco, 1983.
Back Owner's Manual (Patient Information Library Series). Daly City, CA: PAS Publishing, 1977.
The ABC's of Perfect Posture. Chicago: American Medical Association (Dept. of Health Education, 535 N. Dearborn St., IL 60610).

Back Exercises

LONG TERM GOAL: The patient will strengthen abdominal, back, and leg muscles; the patient will stretch hamstring muscles and will increase spinal flexibility;

the patient will achieve correct posture and position of pelvis;

the patient will reduce muscular strain and backache;

the patient will improve circulation and oxygenation of all body tissues thereby improving total body conditioning;

the patient will relax mentally as well as physically;

the patient will increase exercise tolerance and acceptance; and

the patient will continue daily back exercises indefinitely to prevent future episodes of low back pain.

General Considerations:

— **When?** Obtain physician's examination and approval of exercise regimen before beginning.

— **What?** Have a doctor check which exercises are to be done, in what order, how many times, and how often. Exercises should be done regularly at least three times weekly, preferably once or twice daily, as age and general condition permits.

— **How?**
  - Take a warm shower or tub bath to increase circulation, to warm up and loosen tight muscles, and to prevent injury to muscles or back.
  - Do the exercises on a hard floor surface covered with a folded blanket or foam mat.
  - Begin the exercises with slow careful movements. Some discomfort is normal, but refrain from exercises that produce pain until you check again with your doctor. Do the exercises in the order listed below, progressing from simple to complex. Do each exercise only three to four times, resting and breathing deeply for at least 30 seconds between exercises. As tolerance, flexibility, and strength increase, do each exercise six to ten times for an exercise period of 25–30 minutes twice daily.

Simple Beginning Exercises

1) Stand with your back next to a wall, heels about three inches from wall, arms at side, shoulder blades and back of head touching wall. Bend your knees, while pressing the small of your back (lumbar spine) against the wall. Slowly straighten legs, keeping your back as straight as possible. Repeat 3x.

2) Stand erect, while facing and holding on to a table, counter, or chair back. Slowly bend knees, squat for 3 seconds, then straighten to a standing position. Rest. Repeat 3x.

3) Sit on a straight back chair with arms at sides, knees apart. Lean forward until forehead rests between knees and fingers rest on floor. Exhale. Pull back into a sitting position, breathing in deeply and tightening abdominal muscles. Rest. Repeat 3x.

4) Lie on your back, arms at sides, knees bent. Without moving, press spine flat against floor; tighten (contract) abdominal muscles and hold for 3 seconds. Breath normally and *do not hold breath while holding position*. Relax. Repeat this "pelvic tilt" exercise at least 5x. This exercise can also be done while sitting during other times of the day.

5) While in back lying position, bend both knees; bring up 1 at a time and clasp your hands under them. Hold for 5 seconds. In this position, *slowly and gently* rock back and forth from side to side, moving whole body as a single unit. Do not twist neck or back. After 10 seconds, straighten legs, 1 at a time, rest 30 seconds and repeat 2x.

6) Lie on your back with knees bent, feet flat on floor. Breathe deeply and relax. Bending 1 knee at a time, pull leg up to chest, straighten leg upward over head, then lower leg to bent knee position and return to floor. Rest, change legs. Repeat exercise 3x with each leg.

7) Get into crawl position, hands and knees on floor. Breathe in deeply, sucking in your abdomen and humping your back like a cat. Lower your head and look at your knees. Hold for 2 to 3 seconds. Exhale and return to starting position. Repeat 5x.

(After 1 week of doing simple exercises, begin the following more advanced exercises)

Advanced Exercises

8) Lie on your back with knees bent, feet flat. Grasp upper legs and pull your trunk into a sitting position, then lower slowly to the original back lying position; rest. Repeat sit-ups 3–6x.
   - At first have someone hold your feet or anchor them under the edge of a sofa (or other heavy piece of furniture). After a few weeks of practice, you will not need to have your feet held.

9) When exercise 8) can be done easily, progress to a sit-up from a back lying position with legs straight and arms stretched out overhead. Slowly sit, reaching your ankles while pressing your heels and the small of your back into the floor. Avoid quick jerking movements. Count to 8 as you sit up *and* as you return to back lying position. Repeat 3–6x.

10) When exercise 9) can be done easily, do sit-ups with hands clasped behind head.

11) Do this exercise only after first 10 have been done regularly for at least 6–8 weeks.Lie on your back, arms at sides, hands flat on floor under buttocks. Take a deep breath and relax. Bend both legs together, straighten into air as high as comfortable and *slowly* lower legs to floor, pausing momentarily when they are about 10 inches off floor. Keep lumbar region (small of back) pressed into floor. Repeat 5x. When this can be done easily, progress to leg scissors movements while legs are being lowered to floor, holding for at least 5 seconds when legs are about 10 inches from floor.

Recommended References

"Back Care." *NCP Guide #3:41*, 2nd Ed., Nurseco, 1983.

Back Owner's Manual (Patient Information Series). Daly City, CA: PAS Publishing, 1977.

"Getting Back into Good Posture: How to Erase Your Aches," by J. Drapeau. *Nursing 75*, September 1975:63–65.

"How to Avoid That Aching Back," by B. Owen. American *Journal of Nursing*, May 1980:894–897.

Diet: Diarrhea Control

GOAL: The patient will experience reduced irritation of the intestine's mucosal lining, lessened stimulation of intestinal motility, lessened abdominal cramping, a reduced number of loose stools, and a return to health associated with the re-establishment of fluid and electrolyte balance, followed by a return to normal dietary intake and intestinal output.

General Considerations:

— **Dietary treatment** of uncomplicated diarrhea is aimed at achieving the above goals. If vomiting occurs, nothing by mouth is offered until one to two hours after vomiting has ceased. *The physician should be notified* (and hospitalization may be advised) if vomiting persists, if fever is present, if there is blood in the stool, if abdominal pain is severe and steady, if the diarrhea or abdominal pain continues more than 24–48 hours with little or no improvement, if the patient is an infant under six months of age, or elderly, or infirm, or if signs of dehydration are evident. The nurse or parent should observe for decreased urination, lack of saliva, sunken eyeballs, lethargy or listlessness, or absence of tears. Hospitalization for parenteral fluids, electrolytes, and calories along with medications will be needed for acute cases.

— **Principles of dietary management** include:
  • increased calories to compensate for recent losses;
  • increased vitamins and minerals (sodium, potassium, chloride) to counteract losses and diminished absorption;
  • decreased protein, fat, and fiber to give irritated intestines a rest; and
  • slow, gradual resumption of bland, soft foods in small amounts as tolerance, appetite, and stool consistency indicate a normal diet might be resumed without diarrheal recurrence.

Foods and Fluids to be Avoided for at Least a Week:

— Skimmed milk because it contains lactose and presents a high renal solute load (obligating water for urine); boiling increases water loss and sodium content, further complicating situation.
— Bouillon and broth because they are high in sodium and chloride, but low in potassium and glucose. (Edema has been reported in infants given this for diarrhea.)
— Fats (butter, eggs, milk, ice cream, and most cheeses).
— Meats, raw vegetables, spicy foods, pastries, candy, nuts, or gas-forming foods.
— Whole wheat, rye breads, and high-fiber cereals.

Foods and Fluids Recommended (for less severe cases of dehydration and mild diarrhea):
— *First 8–12 hours*: clear fluids in small frequent amounts (30 cc (1 oz) Q15 minutes); give more for fever or high environmental temperatures. Fluids should be cool or lukewarm, not ice cold or hot. Beverage suggestions include water, Gatorade, flat (decarbonated) 7-Up, ginger ale, Bubble-Up, apple juice, popsicles, sweetened weak tea, powdered soft drink mixes, liquid gelatin (twice the recommended water and not allowed to jell).
— *Second 12 hours*: add diluted orange juice and carrot soup (jar of strained carrots with jar of water); for babies, use Lytren or Pedialyte (available in drugstores), which provide appropriate quantitities of all 3 needed electrolytes, as well as glucose.
— *24–48 hours*: add small feedings Q2H of white toast with jelly, rice (plain) or rice cereal, saltine crackers, bananas, pureed *fresh* apples (without skin), plain low-fat yogurt, baked or boiled potato (without butter), broiled white meat of chicken or *lean*, ground beef. Infants may be given their usual full-strength formula if diarrhea has subsided.
— *Third day*: 6 small meals of soups, canned or cooked fruits, and vegetables added to above choices. Infants may be given their usual full-strength formula if diarrhea has subsided.
— *After third or fourth day*: slowly resume normal diet as desired and tolerated, avoiding alcohol, fatty milk products, spicy, high-fiber, or gas-forming foods for several more days.

Recommended References
"Home Care for Diarrhea" (Patient Education Aid). *Patient Care*, March 15, 1981:163.

Diet: Sodium-Restricted

GOAL: The patient will establish and maintain a sodium-restricted diet as prescribed by his physician in order to restore normal sodium balance in the body; the patient will ingest sufficient balanced nutrients to maintain ideal body weight.

General Considerations

— Sodium-restricted diets are calculated to provide *only* the prescribed amount of sodium allowed in the daily diet (250 mg, 500 mg, 1000 mg, or mild sodium restriction) and to provide a well-balanced diet containing proteins, fats, carbohydrates, minerals, and vitamins in proportions necessary to maintain health and ideal body weight. Many patients on a sodium-restricted diet are overweight and put on a low-calorie diet as well.

— **Dietary teaching** is usually done by a dietician and reinforced by nurses. The American Heart Association has developed meal plans for sodium-restricted diets. These are not definitive diets, but a ready-reference guide only, and should be used as such. Be sure to obtain the current AHA diet booklets.

— **Indications** for use of a sodium-restricted diet include liver disease, hypertension, congestive heart failure, and renal disease.

— **Nursing responsibilities** include teaching the patient the basic goals and rationale of sodium-restricted diets as outlined below, providing the patient with resource materials so that s/he can complete own food lists, teaching the patient to plan own menus, critiquing and correcting them PRN, and observing (and teaching) patient for signs of sodium depletion (muscle cramps, convulsions, hypotension, hypovolemia, and poor renal function).

General Rules:

1) Avoid foods that are processed, prepared, or preserved with sodium compounds (salt, MSG, baking powder, baking soda, di-sodium phosphate, sodium alginate, etc.).
2) Read labels carefully for sodium additions and content.
3) Eat only those foods on the diet list, in the amounts given; plan meals carefully.
4) Check the amount of sodium in the drinking water supply. It should contain no more than 5 mg sodium; if it contains more, use distilled water. (Remember, the object is to avoid sodium, rather than just salt.)
5) Be aware that sodium is present in medications such as antibiotics, cough medicines, pain relievers. Rinse mouth well after using toothpaste, mouth washes, since some contain large amounts of sodium.

6) Measure quantities of food carefully using standard measuring cups and spoons; weigh meats.

7) Do not use a salt substitute unless the physician has recommended a specific kind.

8) Experiment with and utilize sodium-free herbs and spices to flavor foods.

The following is from the AHA 500 mg sodium, 1800 calorie plan.

Category	Allowed	To Be Avoided
Milk & Cheese	2 glasses (regular, evaporated, skim, powdered) ⅓ cup *unsalted* cottage cheese 1 ounce low sodium dietetic cheese	Ice cream, sherbert, malted milk, milk shakes, chocolate or condensed milk, regular cottage cheese
Fat	*Unsalted* butter or margarine; *unsalted* cooking fat, oil, french dressing, mayonnaise, nuts	Salted butter, margarine, cooking fat, oil; bacon or ham fat; salt pork; olives, salted nuts, commercial salad dressings
Eggs	1 egg daily	
Meat, Fish, Fowl	Fresh, frozen, or dietetic canned meat or poultry (beef, lamb, pork, veal, fresh tongue, liver, chicken, duck, turkey, rabbit); fresh or dietetic canned (not frozen) fish	Brains or kidneys; canned salted or smoked meat (bacon, bologna, corned or chipped beef, frankfurters, ham, meats koshered by salting, luncheon meats, salt pork, sausage, smoked tongue) Frozen fish fillets; canned, salted or smoked fish, canned tuna or salmon Shellfish (clams, crabs, lobsters, oysters, scallops, shrimp, etc.)
Vegetables	Fresh, frozen, or canned dietary vegetables except those "to be avoided"	Canned vegetables or vegetable juices unless they are low sodium, dietetic Frozen vegetables if processed with salt Artichokes, beet greens, beets, carrots, celery, chard, whole hominy, kale, mustard greens, sauerkraut, spinach, white turnips

Category	Allowed	To Be Avoided
Breads, Cereals, Cereal Products	Low sodium bread, rolls, crackers, *unsalted* melba toast Dry cereals (puffed rice, puffed wheat, shredded wheat) Plain *unsalted* matza Macaroni or noodles, spaghetti, rice, barley *Unsalted* popcorn, flour	Regular breads, crackers Commercial mixes Cooked cereals containing a sodium compound Dry cereals other than those listed or those having more than 6 mg of sodium in 100 gm of cereal Self-rising cornmeal or self-rising flour Potato chips, pretzels, salted popcorn
Fruits	Any fruit or fruit juice (if sugar has not been added)	Fruits canned or frozen in sugar (contain extracalories), dried fruit with sodium sulfate added
Miscellaneous	Coffee (regular & instant), coffee substitutes, tea, lemons, limes, plain unflavored gelatin, vinegar, cream of tartar, potassium bicarbonate, sodium-free baking powder, yeast	Instant cocoa mixes, instant coffee treated with a sodium compound; other beverage mixes, including fruit-flavored powders, fountain beverages, malted milk; soft drinks (both regular and low-calorie); any kind of commercial bouillon (cubes, powders or liquids), sodium cyclamate and sodium saccharin; commercial candies, commercial gelatin desserts; regular baking powder, baking soda (sodium bicarbonate), rennet tablets, molasses, pudding mixes

For 250 mg Na diet, substitute low-Na milk for regular milk.

For 1000 mg Na diet, follow a 500 mg Na diet, and add one of the following for the additional 500 mg:

¼ tsp. salt (scant)   1 cup drained sauerkraut
¾ tsp. monosodium glutamate   1 cup tomato juice
½ bouillon cube   1½ ounces ham
Average serving of cooked cereal, rice, spaghetti,   1 average frankfurter
noodles, hominy, etc. seasoned with salt

Sample Diet Plan for 500 mg sodium, 1800 calorie diet:

Breakfast	**Lunch**	**Dinner**

Breakfast

½ cup orange juice
1 scrambled egg
2 slices low-sodium toast
1 small pat unsalted butter
Coffee or tea ad lib

Lunch

2 ounces broiled liver
⅓ cup fresh peas
Cabbage slaw with caraway seeds, green
    peppers, & vinegar
1 medium low-sodium muffin
1 pat unsalted butter
Apricot bread pudding made with:
   1 slice low-sodium bread
   ¼ cup milk
   4 dried apricot halves
   1 small pat unsalted butter
Coffee or tea ad lib

Dinner

Baked casserole of beef with whipped potato
Topping made with:
   2 oz. cooked beef
   ½ cup broth from beef
   ½ cup potato
Green beans
Tomato, cucumber & lettuce salad with 1 tbsp
    low-sodium French dressing
1 medium low-sodium roll
1 small pat unsalted butter
½ cup mixed fruit
Coffee or tea ad lib

Snacks:

Mid-morning: ½ cup milk, 5 low-sodium crackers
Mid-afternoon: 1 small pear, ¼ cup milk
Evening: 1 small banana, ½ cup milk

Recommended References:

Easy-to-Use Guide to Sodium in Food, Medicine & Water. Lombard, IL: Water Quality Association, (477 E Butterfield Road, 60148).

Handbook of Clinical Dietetics. American Dietetic Association. New Haven: Yale University Press, 1981:G3–G14.

"Helping the Hypertensive Patient Control Sodium Intake," by M. Hill. *American Journal of Nursing.* May 1979:906–909.

"Salt and High Blood Pressure." *Consumer Reports,* March 1979:147–149.

Special Foods and Food Products for Use with Sodium or Salt Restricted Diets. Los Angeles: American Heart Association, 1973.

Your 500 Milligram Sodium Diet, Your 1000 Milligram Sodium Diet, Your Mild Sodium Restricted Diet. New York: American Heart Association (44 E 23rd Street, 10010, or a local
   affiliate).

Drugs: Hypnotics & Sedatives

Definition: Appropriate lower dosages of the below-listed drugs (which are central nervous system depressants) induce relaxation and are called "sedatives;" larger doses induce sleep and are called "hypnotics;" progressively increasing doses cause anesthesia, coma, and death.

GOALS: To sedate, to induce sleep, to reduce anxiety, to suppress convulsions, to produce partial anesthesia or amnesia.

General Considerations:

— **Use of barbiturates** (Class II of Controlled Substances Act) has declined by more than 75% since 1977; *non-barbiturate drugs* now account for more than half of sedative-hypnotic prescriptions. Both types are considered effective for short-term use (two to four weeks), and both carry adverse consequences in long-term use. Either type may be prescribed, depending on a particular patient's need and the cause of the underlying insomnia; long-term use of either is not considered justified.

— **Non-barbiturates,** such as chloral hydrate, paraldehyde, ethinamate, and ethchlorvynol, are usually recommended for patients with impaired liver or renal function and for those who cannot tolerate barbiturates. Elderly patients with organic brain syndrome, alcoholics, and some types of psychotics require close monitoring and careful, judicious use of non-barbiturate drugs. For drug sensitive persons who require low dosages of milder preparations, antihistamines are commonly used as sedative-hypnotics. They are sometimes effective for occasional, at-home, non-prescriptive use.

— **Non-drug treatment of insomnia** includes:
  • discovery of the underlying cause, whether organic, psychiatric, or environmental, and appropriate steps to remove or control cause;
  • assessment of particular patient's sleep pattern and associated habits as well as their own perception of need for a given number of hours of unbroken sleep;
  • identification of pre-sleep activities, including eating, exercise, or mental work, and analysis of facilitative or detrimental effect on sleep inducement; and
  • counseling patient on pre-sleep behaviors that warrant experimental modification. The patient's involvement, cooperation, and acceptance must be solicited. These changes may include:
    — avoiding those foods known to cause indigestion, flatus, or diarrhea;
    — avoiding excessive fluid intake and stimulant drinks such as coffee, tea, chocolate, or cola, as well as alcohol;
    — avoiding late afternoon or early evening naps *if* they are known to interfere with desired nightime sleep;

      — trying one or more activities thought to be relaxing for a particular individual, e.g., hobbies, listening to or playing music, reading, exercise, warm baths, drinking warm milk; and

      — carrying out a stress-reduction regimen on a daily basis.

— **When a patient has a PRN order** for a hypnotic or sedative, assess the patient's real need and behavior, basing the decision to medicate on assessment findings and good judgment; give PRN meds only after this assessment. At the same time, if patients have been taking sedatives at home each night, any attempt to wean them will probably be futile and complicate their condition with withdrawal symptoms. Hospital routine and environment makes effective sleep difficult at best, so if there is no underlying cause for the patient's insomnia that can be dealt with otherwise, hypnotic and sedative administration is usually justified.

•   — **Nursing responsibilities** include:

    1) *teaching* patients and families the correct use of sedative and hypnotic drugs, the dangers of combining other medications, the side effects and toxic effects to note and report;

    2) *employing* a wide variety of nondrug techniques to calm and relax a patient, to help him sleep more restfully, and to cope more effectively with stress (refer to NCPG #5:49, "Stress Management");

    3) *continuing* own pharmacology education in order to know effects of drug interactions and the importance of learning what other medications a patient is taking when hypnotics or sedatives are prescribed;

    4) *safeguarding* drugs to prevent patients from accumulating them; and

    5) *observing and recording* responses to medication, including levels of awareness, vital signs, gastrointestinal symptoms, rashes, etc.

Drug Type & Actions, Examples	Side Effects & Toxic Effects	Nursing Implications

A. Barbiturates
CNS depressants; reduce BP and mental activity; larger doses produce cardiac and respiratory depression.
   amobarbital sodium (Amytal)
   pentobarbital sodium (Nembutal)
   phenobarbital (Luminal, Eskabarb)
   secobarbital (Seconal)
	Skin eruptions, photosensitivity, drowsiness, lethargy, headache, vertigo, diarrhea, excitement, restlessness, euphoria. Overdose, acute toxic effects are slurred speech, ataxia, anoxia, cyanosis, respiratory depression, rapid feeble pulse, decreased body temperature, peripheral vascular collapse, pulmonary edema.	• Observe and record patient responses, complaints; teach patient side effects to report.
		• Check vital signs; maintain adequate airway, administer oxygen, record I&O, prepare for renal or peritoneal dialysis; gastric aspiration and lavage may be done, but do not induce emesis.

Drug Type & Actions, Examples	**Side Effects & Toxic Effects**	**Nursing Implications**
	Habitual usage causes physical and psychological dependence, compulsive use, addiction and withdrawal symptoms of convulsions, and delirium tremens.	• Observe cautious gradual withdrawal while observing patient for anxiety, tremor, weakness, or ECG changes.
	When given with Dilantin, hydrocortisone, griseafulvin, anticoagulants, or butazolidin, barbiturates decrease their effect due to diminished aborption or increased breakdown in liver.	• Know what other meds patient is taking and watch for effects when barbiturate is discontinued or lowered in dosage.
	Effect of barbiturate is enhanced when taken with alcohol, antihistamines, antianxiety drugs, narcotics, phenothiazines, sulfonamides.	• Know what other drugs patient is taking and observe for CNS depression, stupor, coma, respiratory depression. • Teach patient dangers of combining meds at home without MD's knowledge.
B. Non-Barbiturates CNS depressants; little marked effect on cardiac, respiratory, or gastrointestinal activity		• Observe for dependence; caution about dangers of abrupt withdrawal.
chloral hydrate (Aquachloral, Felsules, Lycoral, Noctec, Somnos)	Nausea, vomiting, skin reactions, gastritis, allergic reactions; interacts adversely with anticoagulants (potentiating anticoagulant) and with MAO inhibitors (increasing chloral hydrate effect).	• Measure I&O, reporting changes; observe behavior, inspect skin. Know what other drugs patient is taking; check vital signs QID.
ethchlorvynol (Placidyl)	Hangover, fatigue, drowsiness, giddiness, vertigo, blurred vision, bad aftertaste	• Observe and report all unusual behavior and complaints.
ethinamate (Valmid)	Few untoward reactions; mild GI symptoms, skin rash	• Same as above

Drug Type & Actions, Examples	Side Effects & Toxic Effects	Nursing Implications
paraldehyde (Paral)	Unpleasant odor and taste, nausea, headache, dizziness	• Mix with syrup, fruit juice or milk; serve cold to minimize odor and taste.
methaqualone (Quaalude, Sopor, Somnafac Parest, Optimil)	Headache, hangover, fatigue, tingling & numbness in extremities, dry mouth, anorexia, dizziness, torpor	• Used for withdrawal of drug-addicted patient; make sure that patient does not hoard pills, note carefully face flushing or paleness (signs of intoxication).
Benzodiazepines, Propanediols	Refer to NCPG #3:47, "Drugs: Tranquilizers (Minor)."	

Recommended References

"Drugs: Tranquilizers (Minor)." *NCP Guide #3:47*, 2nd Ed., Nurseco, 1983.
"Hypnotic Drugs and Treatment of Insomnia," by Council on Scientific Affairs, AMA. *Journal of the American Medical Association*, February 1981:749–750.
"Sedative-Hypnotic Drugs," by E. Harris. *American Journal of Nursing*, July 1981:1329–1334.
"Stress Management." *NCP Guide #5:49*, Nurseco, 1981.

Drugs: Psychotropic

Definition: Psychotropic drugs are those that affect the functioning of the mind.

GOAL: To enhance patient contact with reality and to make the patient more accessible to psychotherapy.

General Considerations:
- **Drug dosage** varies according to individual symptoms, severity of mental disturbance, tolerance levels, general health status, and other drugs being used.
- **Nursing responsibilities** include *knowledge* of effect, usual dosage, side effects and nursing implications for each prescribed drug; *administration* of drugs as ordered, verifying with doctor any dose you question as to safety or dosage; *observation* to ensure patient has swallowed drug; *charting* of patient responses and notifying doctor of side effects; and *teaching* patient and significant other as needed in setting and as preparation for discharge.
- **On an in-patient basis,** use PRN sedation as specifically as possible; always make an attempt to find out what prevents the patient from resting or participating in activities and make effort to remedy the situation. Recognizing anxiety and distress in daytime and coping with the problem before it becomes severe is vital. *Take one or more of the following measures before giving PRN sedation or tranquilizers:* encourage patient to remain awake, out of bed, and to exercise in daytime; warm bath; backrub; warm, unstimulating drink; calm and relaxed ward atmosphere; quiet talk or presence of staff member; an extra smoke with supervision; quiet, monotonous occupation before bedtime; eliminate specific discomfort; explore relationship with other patients and staff.
- **On an out-patient basis,** assess patient's method and regularity of taking medications and attitude about them. Ask specifically: how many? what time of day? does s/he ever cut down on medication? what does s/he do if s/he forgets to take dose? Patient may feel that all medications are habituating or not want to be dependent on drugs; the precipitating event to an acute episode is often the patient deciding to discontinue medication.
- **Minor tranquilizers** are useful in the management of acute anxiety and tension; they relieve anxiety better than barbiturates; are palliative, not curative. See NCPG #3:47, "Drugs: Tranquilizers," for specifics.

— **Anti-Parkinsonian drugs** are often given with phenothiazines to prevent extrapyramidal symptoms. They inhibit the parasympathetic nervous system and relax smooth muscle. Examples are trihexyphenidyl (Artane), benztropine (Cogentin), levodopa (Larodopa, Dopar). Side effects include toxic symptoms of blurred vision, vertigo, tachycardia, confusion. Benztropine causes side effects similar to those of atropine, and levodopa may cause nausea, vomiting, hypotension, choreiform movements. The drugs are contraindicated in patients with glaucoma.

Drug Type & Action, Examples
A. Anti-psychotics

The action of this group of drugs is one of lessening the psychotic process and normalizing behavior.

1) *Phenothiazines*: Most effectively used in treatment of schizophrenia; may be beneficial in treatment of other functional psychoses, mania, agitated depression, and behavioral disorders resulting from organic brain disease. Drug effects are similar in this group; specific drug is chosen to increase or decrease side effects.

   chlorpromazine (Thorazine)
   thioridazine (Mellaril)
   fluphenazine (Prolixin)
   penphenazine (Trilafon)
   prochlorperazine (Compazine)
   trifluoperazine (Stelazine)

Side Effects & Toxic Effects

All the antipsychotic drugs produce essentially the same side effects; dangerous ones occur rarely. Side effects may be grouped as *autonomic*: dry mouth, stuffy nose, blurred vision, postural hypotension, constipation; or *extrapyramidal*: (1) *dystonia*—bizarre, involuntary movements of arms, legs, face and neck, often painful; may have difficulty talking & swallowing; onset may be sudden; (2) *Parkinson-like syndrome*—mask-like facies, tremor, rigidity, shuffling gait; (3) *akathisia*—restlessness, often difficult to differentiate from psychotic agitation. *Other:* jaundice; agranulocytosis; allergic skin reactions; photosensitivity; drowsiness; decreased mental alertness; breast engorgement; decreased libido; increased appetite; reduced convulsive threshold. Potentiates alcohol.

Nursing Implications

- Teach patient potential side effects, to be alert to them and to report any occurrence.
- Rinse dry mouth with water; avoid candy, gum, etc. as prolonged use may contribute to dental caries.
- If patient has dizziness or postural hypotension, teach to sit up slowly, pause, and make a gradual change to being upright.
- Reassure that extrapyramidal symptoms are common and usually temporary.
- Advise patient to report fevers or sore throats promptly. Avoid sunlight if photosensitivity or skin discoloration present. May drive car, but use extra caution if experiencing side effects. Explain rationale for avoiding alcohol. With all anti-psychotic drugs, symptoms of psychosis often return when

Drug Type & Action, Examples	Side Effects & Toxic Effects	Nursing Implications
		patient stops taking meds; stress the value of daily meds as ordered.
		• Contraindicated with glaucoma.
		• Use cautiously if history of convulsive disorder or heart disease.
2) *Butyrophenones:* *haloperidol (Haldol)* *fentanyl (Innovar)*	Same effect as phenothiazines but less prone to stimulate appetite, less apt to produce orthostatic hypotension.	• As above; Haldol particularly good for aged patients. May cause depression after manic phase.
3) *Thioxantheses:* *chlorprothixene (Taractan)* *thiothixine (Navane)*	Chemically related to phenothiazines, and have similar effect.	• As above
B. Anti-depressants Chemical agents that help lift depressions; used in conjunction with psychotherapy.	All this group can produce a toxic psychosis; patient becomes confused, disoriented, and may hallucinate.	• Explain to patient that 3–4 weeks are required for onset of action; teach what side effects to be alert for, and to report any to MD/clinic.
		• Contraindicated if history of hypertension. Do not give with psychomotor stimulants, ephedrine, epinephrine, or meperidine (Demerol), or tricyclic drugs.
1) *Monoamine oxidase (MAO) inhibitors* *isocarboxazid (Marplan)* *tranylcypromine (Parnate)* *phenelzine (Nardil)*	A Parnate (or Nardil) and cheese reaction is a hypertensive crisis (severe headache, dizziness, tachycardia, pallor, chills, stiff neck, N&V, fear, restlessness, muscle twitching, chest pain, palpitation) that occurs when patients take Parnate or Nardil and then	• Advise patient not to eat cheese, yogurt, wine, beer, bananas, avocados, yeast products, broad (Fava) beans, chicken livers, or pickled herring (the drugs contain tyramine, which interacts with these foods). Also wise to avoid

Drug Type & Actions, Examples	Side Effects & Toxic Effects	Nursing Implications
	eat cheese; can occur when taking other MAO inhibitors as well; also have adverse reactions with other foods and certain drugs, including the tricyclic drugs.	large amounts of coffee, tea, and chocolate.
2) *Tricyclic drugs (non-enzyme inhibitors):* This group of drugs is also effective in treating phobic symptoms in patients with severe anxiety. *imipramine (Tofranil)* *amitriptyline (Elavil)* *desipramine (Norpramin)* *perphenazine (Triavil)* *doxepin (Sinequan—although not a tricyclic drug per se, effect is similar.)*	Blurred vision, dry mouth, ataxia, postural hypotension, tachycardia, palpitation, dizziness, fainting, N&V, urinary retention, inability to sleep; profuse sweating, aggravation of glaucoma; stimulates CNS; potentiates alcohol. In large doses, has a sedative action, thus reducing need for sedatives at night. May cause confusion, especially in elderly.	• Patient will usually develop a tolerance to any side effects. Monitor pulse and BP for irregularities. If postural hypotension present, instruct patient to sit up slowly, pause, and make a gradual change to being upright. Check urinary output and BMs daily. Ensure adequate fluid intake. Check with drug manufacturers for incompatible drugs. A dose of 50–100 tabs can be lethal; limit amount a patient has at any one time. • Contraindicated before surgery or with history of glaucoma, epilepsy, congestive heart failure.
3) *CNS Stimulants:* Give feeling of energy and well-being; used to treat mild depression. Chemical and biological similarity to ephedrine and amphetamine. *methylphenidate (Ritalin)* *dextroamphetamine (Dexedrine)* *methamphetamine (Methedrine)*	Tachycardia, hypertension, dry mouth, headache, jitteriness, insomia, decreased appetite; increased susceptibility to accidents, addiction. Nervousness & insomnia; overcomes drug-induced lethargy caused by tranquilizers. High drug abuse potential; masks warning signs of fatigue. Anorexia & weight loss, especially in children.	• Advise patient of potential side effects and observe for same; reduce dosage with side effects. • Teach safety precautions. Avoid using with dependent type persons. • Check for potentiation of other drugs and discuss with MD.

4) *Lithium carbonate:* Normalizes pathologic mood without sedation or impairment of intellectual functioning. Is used to treat acute mania and to prevent recurring manic-depressive episodes. Blood levels must be maintained within a narrow range.

Minor side effects include fine tremor, nausea, diarrhea, ataxia, drowsiness, thirst, polyuria.

Moderate side effects include nausea and vomiting, ataxia, dizziness, slurred speech, blurred vision, increasing tremor, muscle irritability or twitching.

Toxic symptoms include severe tremor, marked drowsiness, confusion, nystagmus, oliguria, chorea, convulsions.

- Requires 1–2 weeks for onset of action. Most patients experience some temporary side effects.
- Reassure patient that tremor is common, non-hazardous and will disappear. If patient nauseated, instruct to take pills with meals.
- Teach family potential side effects, to observe for signs of increasing untoward ones, and to report to MD.
- Coordinate arrangements for monitoring patient's serum lithium levels (done weekly initially, then usually bi-monthly for maintenance).
- Be especially alert to side effects/toxic symptoms in patients on diuretics, on a low salt diet, thyroid extract, or those with impaired renal function or CHF.

Recommended References

"Antidepressant Drug Therapy," by M. DeGennaro et al. *American Journal of Nursing*, July 1981:1304–1310.

"Antipsychotic Medications," by E. Harris. *American Journal of Nursing*, July 1981:1316–1319.

"Drug Interactions and Altered Actions in Psychopharmacology," by D.D. Gold, Jr. *Hospital Formulary*, March 1981:313–316.

"Drugs: Hypnotics & Sedatives." *NCP Guide #3:45*, 2nd Ed., Nurseco, 1983.

"Drugs: Parkinson's Disease." *NCP Guide #2:38*, 2nd Ed., Nurseco, 1980.

"Drugs: Tranquilizers." *NCP Guide #3:46*, 2nd Ed., Nurseco, 1983.

"Extrapyramidal Side Effects of Antipsychotic Therapy," by E. Harris. *American Journal of Nursing*, July 1981:1324–1328.

"Lithium," by Elizabeth Harris. *American Journal of Nursing*, July 1981:1310–1315.

"Manic-Depression: An Overview," by D.L. Divson. *Journal of Psychiatric Nursing*, June 1981:28–31.

"Medication Group for Psychiatric Patients," by M. Cohen et al. *American Journal of Nursing*, February 1981:343–345.

"Nursing Care of Patients on Lithium," by S. Hunn et al. *Perspectives in Psychiatric Care*, September/October 1980:214–220.

"Preventing Excessive Weight Gain from Psychotropic Drugs." *Nurses Drug Alert*, January 1981:5.

"Preventing Psychotropic-Induced Seizures." *Nurses Drug Alert*, March 1981:23.

"Psychotropic Drug Use and Polypharmacy in a General Hospital," by C. Salzman. *General Hospital Psychiatry*, March 1981:1–9.

"Psychotropic Usage in Long-term Care Facility Geriatric Patients," by J.W. Cooper et al. *Hospital Formulary*, April 1981:407–409.

"A Study of Antipsychotic Drug Use in Nursing Homes," by W.A. Ray et al. *American Journal of Public Health*, May 1980:485–491.

"Vitamin C Replacement—Fluphenazine Interaction." *Nurses Drug Alert*, November 1979:131.

"When a Patient on Lithium is Pregnant," by H.A. Birgess. *American Journal of Nursing*, November 1979:1989–1992.

Drugs: Tranquilizers (Minor)

GOAL: To reduce anxiety and tension, to relax skeletal muscles, to prevent convulsions, to sedate, to induce sleep, to serve as an adjunct to anesthesia, or to control alcohol-withdrawal symptoms.

General Considerations:
— **Stress and anxiety** are usual concomitants of hospitalization; minor tranquilizers are very useful in alleviating tension without the severe sedative effect seen in barbiturates. Compared to the latter, tranquilizers produce less CNS and respiratory depression, and there is a wider safety margin between therapeutic and toxic doses.
— **Each patient should be evaluated individually** re: need for tranquilizers, the appropriate type and dosage, the likelihood of self-medication with increased dosage. Re-evaluation for response and effectiveness should be made at regularly scheduled intervals (two to six weeks) before continuing medication. Withdrawal regimen should be gradual and closely monitored.
— **An overdose** of a minor tranquilizer can put the patient into a coma, but it is usually not lethal, unless ingested with alcohol, narcotics, or other sedatives. Intravenous fluids with medications to counteract hypotension and CNS depression are given STAT along with gastric lavage or emesis induction.
— **Nursing responsibilities** include:
  1) teaching patients and families the correct use of tranquilizers, the dangers of combining with other medications, and the side and toxic effects to note and report;
  2) employing a wide variety of nondrug techniques to calm and relax a patient, to help him sleep more restfully, and to cope more effectively with stress (refer to NCPG #5:49, "Stress Management");
  3) exercising judgment and discretion with PRN orders (based on assessment of need, not just expediency);
  4) safeguarding drugs to prevent patients from accumulating them;
  5) observing, recording, and reporting responses to medication; and
  6) continuing own pharmacology education to know effects of drug interactions with tranquilizers.
— Refer to NCPG #3:46, "Drugs: Psychotropic," for information on the major tranquilizers, phenothiazines, and others and to NCPG #3:45, "Hypnotics and Sedatives."

Drug Type & Actions, Examples

A. Propanediols

Skeletal muscle relaxant, anti-anxiety
meprobamate (Equanil, Miltown)

tybamate (Solacen, Tybatran)

B. Benzodiazepines

CNS depressant, anti-anxiety, anticon-
vulsant, skeletal muscle relaxant
chlordiazepoxide (Librium)
clorazepate dipotassium (Tranxene)
clorazepate monopotassium (Azene)
clonazepam (Clonopin)
diazepam (Valium)
flurazepam (Dalmane)
lorazepam (Ativan)
oxazepam (Serax)
prazepam (Verstran)

Side Effects & Toxic Effects

Drowsiness, lethargy, slurred speech, ataxia, paradoxical excitement, physical and
psychological dependence, compulsive
use

Same as above, plus dry mouth, glossitis,
confusion, lightheadedness

Sedation, lowered BP, dizziness, fatigue,
ataxia, drowsiness. Less frequently: confusion, depression, headache, nausea,
incontinence, depression, paradoxical excitement or sleep disorders
Serious, but rare: jaundice, skin rashes,
bone marrow depression
Withdrawal symptoms: N&V, anxiety, irritability, seizures

Nursing Implications

- Warn patient to avoid operating dangerous machinery.
- Teach patient dangers of combining
  with alcohol, narcotics, or other
  sedatives.
- Encourage mouth rinsing & extra fluid
  intake.

- Check vital signs QID.
- Observe and record behavioral
  responses.
- Same as above re: operation of machinery.
- Observe for postural hypotension; if
  present, teach patient to sit up slowly,
  pause, and make a gradual change to
  being upright.
- Observe skin color, condition; withhold
  drug, report to MD.
- Observe and closely monitor gradual
  withdrawal of medication.
- Carefully supervise patient intake of ex-
  act dosage; prevent hoarding.

Drug Type & Actions, Examples	Side Effects & Toxic Effects	Nursing Implications
C. Diphenylmethane Derivative Mildly sedative, tranquilizer, antiemetic, antispasmodic *hydroxyzine (Atarax, Vistaril)*	Drowsiness, dry mouth, involuntary motor activity (tremors), convulsions. Can cause birth defects. Reports of tissue irritation with injections	• Warn female patients not to take tranquilizers during pregnancy, if possible. • Same as above for other tranquilizers. • Use "Z" track technique for IM injections.

Recommended References
"Drugs: Hypnotics and Sedatives." *NCP Guide #3:45*, 2nd Ed., Nurseco, 1983.
"Drugs: Psychotropic." *NCP Guide #3:46*, 2nd Ed., Nurseco, 1983.
"Sedatives—Hypnotic Drugs," by E. Harris. *American Journal of Nursing*, July 1981:1329–1334.
"Stress Management." *NCP Guide #5:49*, Nurseco, 1981.
"The Use of Antianxiety Drugs," by F. Berger. *Clinical Pharmacology and Therapeutics*, March 1981:291–293.
"What to Watch for with Minor Tranquilizers," by S. White and K. Williamson. *RN*, November 1979:57–59.

Fluids & Electrolytes: Part A—Fluids

GOAL: The patient will maintain homeostasis, free of preventable fluid imbalances; fluid imbalance will be detected promptly and corrected adequately.

General Considerations:
— **Body fluid and electrolyte imbalances are common to a number of illnesses** and each seriously ill patient has the potential for one or more of these imbalances. Because of the interrelationship, read NCPG #3:49, "Electrolytes."
— **Fluids and electrolytes are gained and lost from the body in various ways.** Fluid *intake* is accomplished orally (by ingestion of food and liquids), IV, NG tube, and as a product of metabolism of food and tissue breakdown (300–500 ml/day). Fluid *losses* are categorized as: (1) *sensible* (or measurable) (a) urine: 600 ml/24 hours output is required to clear a normal solute load and to prevent an increase in BUN, creatinine, and other solutes excreted by the kidney; (b) stool: 10–200 ml water per 24 hours; and (c) other: daily losses from drain sites, diarrhea, emesis, NG tube, renal losses due to complications of diuretic therapy or renal disease; (2) *insensible* (or not measurable) from lungs and skin: 850–1000 ml per 24 hours for an average adult. Insensible losses increase in hyperventilation, sweating, and by 7% per degree F elevation of body temperature above 98.6°.
— **Fluids and electrolytes move within the body in three main ways:** (1) *diffusion*: particles in solution tend to spread uniformly throughout solution across cell membranes *from an area of higher concentration to an area of lower concentration* of solute until a state of equilibrium is reached; (2) *filtration*: fluid movement across cell membranes controlled by hydrostatic pressure (the force exerted by the weight of a solution; mm Hg) will move from *an area of high pressure to an area of low pressure*; and (3) *osmosis*: fluid movement across cell membranes controlled by solute concentration will move from *an area of low solute concentration to an area of high solute concentration* until a state of equilibrium of solute and solvent concentration is reached on both sides of the membrane.
— **Osmolality** reflects the number or concentration of osmotically active solute particles (ions) per weight or kilogram of solvent, and is equal in both extracellular and intracellular compartments. Normal plasma or serum osmolality is about 290–300 mOsm (milliosmoles) per liter. Ions act to maintain osmolality and exist in dynamic equilibrium.
— **There are two main divisions or compartments of body fluids:** (1) *extracellular (ECF)* includes plasma (5% of body weight) and interstitial water surrounding the cells (15% of body weight); (2) *intracellular (ICF)* is the volume of water *within* cells (40% body weight). Note: the percentage of body weight representing total body water (60%) is higher in males than females (females have proportionally more fat).

— **Regulatory mechanisms of fluid and electrolytes:** cations and anions exert osmotic pressure that determines the volume of total body water and its distribution between the extracellular and the intracellular compartments. Osmolality is controlled by anti-diuretic hormone (ADH) and volume is controlled by aldosterone. With loss of ECF and a rise in serum osmolality, ADH (from the hypothalamus) is released to increase reabsorption of water at the distal renal tubule; when osmolality is returned to normal, ADH release is inhibited. With decreased vascular volume and perfusion pressure, receptors in the renin-angiotensin system of the kidney effect the release of aldosterone (from the adrenal cortex). Aldosterone enhances renal tubular absorption of sodium and water to increase intravascular volume.

— **Nursing responsibilities** include observing the patient for signs and symptoms of fluid and/or electrolyte imbalance, assessing the patient's hydration status, initiating appropriate nursing actions, and notifying the physician of changes in patient's status.

— **Assessment of a patient's hydration status** includes obtaining a history (both on admission and on a continuing basis) and involves getting answers to these questions:
  - Can the patient's illness affect his fluid balance? How?
  - Does patient have an existing heart condition? (If yes, s/he will be more prone to fluid overload.)
  - Are there any signs and symptoms that seem to fit together? Are there any supporting lab data?
  - Is the patient receiving any medications or treatment that can affect his fluid balance?
  - Is the patient taking adequate fluids by mouth? If not, is patient on IVs?
  - Is the patient losing an excess amount of fluids via vomiting, diarrhea, NG or other drainage tube, excessive perspiration, etc.? What is patient's 24-hour output (sensible measurement + insensible estimate)?

— **Fluid imbalances** are detected by the clinical condition and history of the patient. Common imbalances are:

	ECF Excess	ECF Deficit
Also Known As	Overhydration, fluid volume excess or overload, hypervolemia	Dehydration, hypovolemia
Common Causes	Excessive IV and/or PO fluid intake. (Occurs most commonly because the kidneys are malfunctioning, as a result of CHF, renal or liver disease. A patient with normal heart and kidney function can tolerate an ECF excess quite well, but one with poorly functioning heart or kidneys cannot.)	GI losses (vomiting, diarrhea, fistulous drainage, excessive tap water enemas, loss of intestinal juices, intestinal obstruction). Other causes include decreased water intake, third space accumulation, systemic infection, burns, ascites, or overzealous use of diuretics.

	ECF Excess	**ECF Deficit**
Signs & Symptoms	Dyspnea, acute weight gain (more than 5% of body weight), edema (pitting edema is always a sign of excess ECF), moist rales, increased BP and CVP, engorged neck veins, and tachycardia	Dry skin and mucous membranes, longitudinal wrinkles or furrows on tongue, weight loss (5% of usual body weight), lethargy, change in postural BP, poor skin turgor, decreased fullness of neck veins, N&V, anorexia, oliguria (in severe cases)
Lab Findings	Decreased RBC count, HCT, and Hgb	Increased RBC count, HCT, and Hgb
Treatment Measures	Treatment of underlying cause(s); restriction of Na & fluid intake; diuretics	Correct underlying cause(s) and replace the fluid.

Nursing Responsibilities

ECF Excess:
- Avoid rapid infusion of IVs.
- Measure I&O & body weight accurately and record.
- Observe for edema & signs of dyspnea; (patient in supine position can have increase of 4–8 liters of fluid without detectable edema).
- Monitor vital signs; compare BP readings for significant changes.
- When patient on diuretics, know & observe for signs & symptoms of K depletion (see NCPG #2:48), elevated BUN, metabolic alkalosis (see NCPG #3:40).
- Observe neck veins for distension.
- Report abnormal lab results to MD.

ECF Deficit:
- Maintain accurate I&O, including GI losses, diaphoresis & linen changes (each episode of diaphoresis with necessary linen change may equal loss of 1 liter of ECF).
- Record vital signs and observe for changes.
- Know that some conditions may lead to ECF deficit, such as shock, oliguria, renal failure.
- Observe for fluid accumulation in third space areas (weight gain due to third space accumulation should not be identified as an increase in ECF as this fluid cannot be drawn back into circulation and therefore is considered lost).
- Report abnormal lab results to MD.

ICF Excess

ICF Deficit (can occur ONLY following ECF deficit)

	ICF Excess	**ICF Deficit**
Common Causes	Renal disease, excessive water intake, inappropriate antidiuretic hormone action	Unavailability of water, inability to swallow, loss of an excessive amount of water

	ECF Excess	**ECF Deficit**
Signs & Symptoms	CNS effects such as mental confusion, headache, muscle twitching, coma and convulsions; increased intracranial pressure, lassitude, and weakness; increased BP and body weight; decreased urinary output	Weakness, restlessness, delirium, hyperpnea, flushed skin, elevated temperature, oliguria
Lab Findings	Serum Na *below* 130 mEq/L; serum osmolality below normal; urine hypertonic to plasma	Serum Na *above* 145 mEq/L, elevated plasma protein and urinary specific gravity
Treatment Measures	Restrict fluid intake and correct the underlying cause(s).	Replace water and correct the contributing cause(s).
Nursing Responsibilities	• Measure I&O, body weight accurately & record. monitor vital signs; compare body weight & vital signs with previous readings & check for changes. • Restrict fluids as ordered & regulate IVs. • Observe for CNS symptoms & changes in sensorium. • Report abnormal serum Na level to MD.	• Measure I&O, body weight accurately & record. • Monitor vital signs. • Observe for CNS symptoms. • Report abnormal lab reports to MD.

Recommended References

"Acid-Base Balance." *NCP Guide #3:40*, 2nd Ed., Nurseco, 1983.

Fluids and Electrolytes: A Practical Approach, 2nd Ed., by C.V. Strout, C. Lee, & C. Schaper. Philadelphia: Davis, 1977.

"Fluids and Electrolytes: Part B—Electrolytes." *NCP Guide #3:49*, 2nd Ed., Nurseco, 1983.

Fluids and Electrolytes with Clinical Applications," 2nd Ed., by J. Kee. New York: Wiley, 1978.

"I.V. Fluids and Electrolytes: How to Head off the Risks," by S. White. *RN*, November 1979:60–63.

Nurses' Handbook of Fluid Balance, 2nd Ed., by N. Metheney & W. Snively Jr. Philadelphia: Lippincott, 1974.

"Perioperative Fluids & Electrolytes," by N. Metheney & W. Snively Jr. *American Journal of Nursing*, May 1978:840–844.

"Potassium Imbalance." *NCP Guide #2:49*, 2nd Ed., Nurseco, 1980.

"Symposium on Fluid, Electrolyte, and Acid-Base Balance." *Nursing Clinics of North America*, September 1980:535–646.

"Test Your Knowledge of Fluid and Electrolyte Management," by E. Nicksic. *Nursing 82*, Part I: May 1982:129–135; Part II: June 1982:113–118.

"What's Behind That I.V. Line?" by J. Keithley and K. Traulini. *Nursing 82*, March 1982:33–45.

Fluids & Electrolytes: Part B—Electrolytes

GOAL: The patient will be free of preventable electrolyte imbalances; electrolyte imbalance(s) will be detected promptly and corrected adequately.

General Considerations:
— Read this section in NCPG #3:48, "Fluids."
— **Electrolytes are electrically charged ions** found in both ECF and ICF. Positively charged ions are called *cations*; negatively charged ions are called *anions*. *Sodium* is the major cation in ECF; *potassium* is the major cation in ICF.
— **Electrolytes are expressed in milliequivalents** (mEq) since it is the equivalent weight (or the weight) that will neutralize an ion with a single opposite charge: e.g., Na has a single positive (+) charge and will neutralize Cl, which has a single negative (–) charge. It is also the equivalent weight that determines the number of molecules in solution of both anions and cations. Calcium (Ca) has a valence of two or a double + charge, and will neutralize two molecules with a single negative charge, e.g., chloride (Cl), or one molecule with a double negative charge, e.g., sulphate (SO_4), resulting in calcium chloride ($CaCl_2$) or calcium sulphate ($CaSO_4$).
— **The principle electrolytes and their normal concentration in ECF** are (lab values may vary with lab):

Cations (mEq/L)			Anions (mEq/L)		
Sodium	Na^+	142	Chloride	Cl^-	103
Potassium	K^+	5	Bicarbonate	HCO_3^-	27
Calcium	Ca^{++}	5	Phosphate	HPO_4^-	2
Magnesium	Mg^{++}	3	Sulfate	SO_4^-	1
		155	Organic Acid		6
			Protein		16
					155

— **In intracellular fluid,** Na concentration is approximately 12 mEq/L; K = 155 mEq/L. Phosphate is the most abundant anion.
— **Other normal lab values include:**

BUN	10 -20 mg.%
Creatine	0.5- 1.5 mg.%
Uric Acid	2.5- 8.0 mg.%
Protein	6.0- 8.0 mg.%

— **Common electrolyte imbalances** are those involving sodium, potassium, and calcium.

   1) **Sodium** (Na⁺)

• The average adult ingests 6 gm Na/day; the minimum daily need is 2 gm; any excess is normally excreted through the skin and kidneys.

• A major characteristic of Na is its ability to retain water. Its primary function in the body is to regulate the relationship of body fluids, both the ICF and the ECF. Since the ICF accounts for two-thirds of total body fluid, an alteration in the serum Na level reflects an ICF problem, rather than an ECF one.

• A serum Na level is a reading of the *concentration* of Na in the blood, not the actual amount of Na. This concentration varies with ICF volume, but the actual amount of Na in the body remains the same.

• Na *controls* maintenance of the ECF volume, *regulates* the shift of water between compartments, and *influences* the excretion of water by means of reabsorption. It also *helps regulate* acid-base balance and is an important factor in nerve conduction.

	Na⁺ Excess (Hypernatremia)	Na⁺ Deficit (Hyponatremia)
Common Causes	Often caused by excessive water losses that do not change the Na level in the body but do concentrate it, thus reflecting excess. History usually includes decreased water intake, excessive ingestion of NaCl, prolonged and profuse diarrhea, excessive loss of water through lungs (may be due to a high fever and rapid breathing), prolonged use of potent diuretics.	Either decreased intake or increased output of *Na,* or increased intake or decreased concentrate output of *water*. History includes excessive sweating, drinking of plain (electrolyte-free) water, infusion of electrolyte-free IV, GI losses, repeated water enemas, use of a potent diuretic. Often associated with heat exhaustion, renal disease, low Na diets, burns.
Signs & Symptoms	When the *serum Na reading is increased* & water is lost, symptoms include: dry, sticky mucous membranes, flushed	If deficit is severe, patient may have hypotension, a rapid thready pulse, cold clammy skin, and cyanosis. If

Na⁺ Excess (Hypernatremia)

skin, intense thirst, oliguria; may also have elevated temperature and tachycardia; skin turgor normal. When the *actual amount of Na is increased*, water is often increased (because of Na's ability to hold water); then symptoms are essentially the same as for an ECF excess.

Na⁺ Deficit (Hyponatremia)

both water and Na are deficient, patient will also have signs and symptoms of an ECF deficit. If only Na is lost,
and not water, signs and symptoms will be as for an ECF excess.

Lab Findings

Serum Na level above 150 mEq/L, urine specific gravity above 1.030 (with a water deficit); this lab reading may be low or unchanged if there is a combined problem. Elevated RBC, hematocrit, plasma protein, BUN, serum osmolality, and urine volume

Serum Na level below 137 mEq/L (indicates a water excess). If both Na and water are lost, there will be no change in serum Na level. Urine specificgravity will be below 1.010 (indicates that the Na in the ECF is decreased); elevated hematocrit, RBC, and plasma protein.

Treatment Measures

When there is an increase in both Na and water, treat like an ECF excess—usually with diuretics and restriction of Na and fluid intake. *When only the Na level is increased*, this reflects an ICF deficit; treat with water replacement, orally or IV.

When there is a loss of both Na and water, treatment is same as for an ECF deficit, usually with an IV of isotonic or hypertonic saline solution. *If only Na is lost*, an ICF excess is indicated; treatment is to restrict fluids.

Nursing Responsibilities

- Assess if patient has an actual or real Na increase, and/or a water excess; know the S&S & treatment for each.
- Measure, chart, and observe for changes in body weight, fluid volume, vital signs.
- Maintain an accurate I&O record.
- Restrict Na intake as ordered.

- Assess if patient has only a Na loss or a loss of both Na and water; know the S&S of ECF deficit & excess.
- Maintain an accurate I&O record.
- Observe for and chart changes in S&S following treatment.

2) **Potassium (K⁺)**
- Deficit (Hypokalemia) and
- Excess (Hyperkalemia): see NCPG #2:48, "Potassium Imbalance."

3) **Calcium (Ca^{++})**
- Ca is important to neuromuscular irritability (has a sedative effect on cell membranes of the nervous system), to normal heart beat, to formation of bones and teeth, and to blood clotting.
- The Ca level in the blood is controlled by parathyroid hormonal activity.
- Ca needs to be ingested each day as it is excreted in the urine and feces. Adequate protein and Vitamin D are essential for the proper utilization of calcium. Nutritional need = 800 mg–1 gm daily.
- Only ionized Ca is physiologically active (½ of serum Ca).
- 90% of Ca in the body is in the bones. When bone is not under stress (i.e., used), decalcification occurs and Ca is lost (rationale behind early ambulation and weight-bearing).

	Ca^{++} Excess (Hypercalcemia)	**Ca^{++} Deficit (Hypocalcemia)**
Common Causes	Often associated with pathologic fractures & renal disease (when Ca cannot be properly excreted); tumor of or hyperactive parathyroid glands, excessive intake of Vit. D, multiple myeloma, prolonged immobility (Ca moves from the teeth & bones to the blood; may result in kidney stones).	Caused by insufficient intake of Ca & Vit. D, malabsorption of Ca from the GI tract, or an excessive loss of Ca, as in renal insufficiencyor hypoparathyroidism. History includes hypoactive or surgical removal of parathyroid glands, sprue, excessive ingestion of citrated blood, massive SC infections (extraction of Ca from ECF), generalized peritonitis, excessive diarrhea, pancreatic disease, stress, diuretic phase of renal failure.
Signs & Symptoms	Hypotonicity of muscles, kidney stones, polyuria, GI symptoms (anorexia, N&V, thirst, constipation); pain in flank, deep bones, and bone cavities. When excess is severe, patient may become lethargic, psychotic, & comatose due to depression of CNS (if Ca level is about 15%).	Tingling of ends of fingers, tetany, abdominal &/or muscle cramps, carpopedal spasms (lack of Ca causes fiber membranes to become partially charged), convulsions, bleeding, prolonged QT interval on ECG
Lab Findings	Serum Ca level above 5.8 mEq/L (10.5mg%); heavy urine precipitation	Serum Ca below 4.5 mEq/L (8.5mg%)

	Ca^{++} Excess (Hypercalcemia)	Ca^{++} Deficit (Hypocalcemia)
Treatment	Aimed at the cause(s) of the excess. IVs and diuretics may be given to encourage renal excretion of Ca; IV or oral phosphate may be given (when phosphorous level is elevated, Ca is excreted through the kidneys); steroids may be given to inhibit the absorption of Ca. If patient is on digitalis, dosage needs to be decreased because Ca excess enhances digitalis intoxication. Ca excess may be decreased with ambulation (pushing Ca back into bones) and corrected by parathyroid surgery. ED-TA IV has been used to chelate calcium & increase renal excretion.	Treat underlying disorder; oral or IV calcium usually given. Vit. D is sometimes given to increase absorption of Ca from the GI tract. For severe tetany, 10–20 ml of 10% Ca gluconate IV is sometimes given.
Nursing Responsi-bilities	• Prevent renal calculi by ensuring mobility whenever possible; otherwise, provide passive exercises QD (see NCPG #2:45, "Hazards of Immobility"), frequent turnings, and a tilt table x 3 daily (weight-bearing). • Increase oral intake to 3–4000 cc QD (unless contraindicated) to dilute the urine & counteract the dehydrating effects of hypercalcemia. • Strain urine for kidney stones. • Observe for and chart CNS and musculoskeletal changes. • Integrate a low Ca diet as ordered into patient's usual dietary habits. • Give patient 250 cc of cranberry or prune juice QD to maintain an acid urine.	• Observe for, chart, and report neuromuscular changes. • Institute seizure precautions; reduce stimuli as much as possible. • Observe patient carefully after giving digitalis (a Ca deficit weakens cardiac muscle contraction). • Keep a tracheotomy tray nearby. • Health-teach patient re: diet & the necessity of eating Ca-containing foods to prevent hypocalcemia and osteoporosis; assess patient's usual use of laxatives and antacids; excessive use may be precipitant to a Ca deficit.

Ca⁺⁺ Excess (Hypercalcemia)

- If on digitalis, know and observe for signs and symptoms of toxicity.
- Be aware that patients with long-standing hypercalcemia may be having a great deal of bone pain, and have a tendency to develop pathological fractures; handle carefully and gently.

Ca⁺⁺ Deficit (Hypocalcemia)

Recommended References

"Electrolyte Solutions: Monitor, Monitor, Monitor," by L. Juliani. *RN*, July 1981:48–49.

"IV Fluids & Electrolytes: How to Head off the Risks," by S. White. *RN*, November 1979:60–63.

Fluids & Electrolytes: A Practical Approach, 2nd Ed., by V. Strout, C. Lee, & C. Schaper. Philadelphia: Davis, 1977.

Fluids & Electrolytes with Clinical Applications, 2nd Ed., by J. Kee. New York: Wiley, 1978.

"Perioperative Fluids & Electrolytes," by N. Metheney and W. Snively Jr. *American Journal of Nursing*, May 1978:840–844.

"Potassium Imbalance." *NCP Guide #2:49*, 2nd Ed., Nurseco 1980.

"Symposium on Fluid, Electrolyte and Acid-Base Balance." *Nursing Clinics of North America*, September 1980:535–646.

"Test Your Knowledge of Fluid and Electrolyte Management," by E. Nicksic. *Nursing 82*, Part I: May 1982:129–135; Part II: June 1982:113–118.

"Understanding the Electrolyte Maze," by Linda Felver. *American Journal of Nursing*, September 1980:1591–1595.

"What's Behind That I.V. Line?" by J. Keithley and K. Traulini. *Nursing 82*, March 1982:33–45.

Hyperalimentation

Definition: Infusion of hypertonic solutions of dextrose, nitrogen, and additives (vitamins, minerals, electrolytes) into a central vein, preferably the superior vena cava.

LONG TERM GOAL: To fulfill the body's energy needs, to achieve a positive nitrogen balance, and to maintain immuno-competence.

General Considerations:
— **Hyperalimentation is frequently given to patients with severe malnutrition or protein loss,** as in gastrointestinal illness (such as malabsorption syndrome, ulcerative colitis), major body burns, large wound infections, carcinoma (especially when the patient is being treated with radiation or chemotherapy), acute renal failure, and central nervous system dysfunction.
— **The procedure** involves three aspects:
   1) **Preparing the solution:** this is done by a registered pharmacist using strict aseptic technique under a laminar flow hood, since the hyperalimentation solution is a fine medium for bacterial and fungal growth. Each bottle is labeled identifying the patient's name, components of solution, and solution's expiration date (not to exceed 24 hours). The standard liter provides 250 gm dextrose (25%), six gm nitrogen, plus electrolytes, vitamins, and minerals according to individual needs as determined by lab tests. The solution is kept refrigerated and brought to room temperature before administering it to the patient.
   2) **Placing the catheter:** a large (#14) intracatheter is inserted infraclavicularly by an MD into the subclavian vein. During insertion, the patient is in Trendelenburg position (makes subclavian easier to reach, increases venous pressure, dilates vessels, and assists in preventing air emboli) and is performing the Valsalva maneuver (bearing down with mouth closed assists in preventing air emboli by increasing intrathoracic pressure and thus the central venous pressure). Have the patient practice the Valsalva maneuver before insertion. Reassure the patient that s/he will experience some pressure in chest during insertion. X-ray confirms location before solutions are administered. A dry, air-occlusive aseptic dressing is placed on the site and changed Q48 hours.
   3) **Giving the solution:** inspect the bottle carefully for cracks and solution clarity. Start infusion slowly (usually one liter QD) and gradually increase to amount needed (two to four liter QD). Administer solution continuously: replace one bottle by another at a steady drip. If delivery is ahead of schedule, add 20% D/W to keep system open.
— **Nursing responsibilities** include emotional and physical preparation of the patient, strict sepsis control, maintenance of the IV system, observation of patient for common complications of catheterization (pneumothorax, artery laceration, phrenic or brachial plexis nerve injury, mediastinal hematoma), and charting pertinent information.

Specific Considerations, Potential Patient Outcomes and Nursing Actions:

1) Prevention of Infection

The patient will be monitored for early signs of infection; strict aseptic technique will be carried out to prevent contamination of the puncture site, catheter, tubing, and/or solution:

— change dressing Q48H, using strict aseptic no-touch technique, sterile gloves & supplies; follow hospital protocol for procedure; apply an air-occlusive dressing;

— assign same nurse to do dressing change in order to decrease chance of contamination & to allow for continuing observations of insertion site by same person for signs of inflammation, swelling, &/or drainage (in many hospitals, dressings are done by the IV nurse);

— change tubing Q24H (should coincide with expiration of current day's supply to eliminate added break in system);

— notify MD & terminate the solution immediately if unexplained temperature spike occurs (add 20% D/W to keep vein open);

— never use infusion line for piggy-back infusion, CVP monitoring, blood withdrawal, or other procedures;

— never irrigate IV catheter.

2) Maintenance of System

The catheter will be maintained in correct position; the infusion will proceed safely and accurately at the prescribed rate; the patient will be monitored for early signs of impending complications:

— caution pt. against scratching or pulling back the tape (hyperalimentation solution & dressing are irritating to skin);

— check IV Q1–2H to prevent & control alterations in infusion; maintain solutions at constant uniform rate; *do not catch up*;

— check tubing for kinks or loose connections;

— observe the following *at least Q4H & PRN* & report any untoward signs to MD:

   • check solution for *turbidity &/or sediment* (notify pharmacist if any found)

   • check vital signs & report any *temperature elevation, dyspnea, or shortness of breath*

   • check urine for S&A to determine *sugar overload* (greater than 3 requires a blood sugar determination)

   • observe *complaints of pain or swelling in shoulder and neck* (may indicate infiltration or thrombosis)

   • observe pt. for signs of *circulatory overload* (prominence of neck veins, shortness of breath, edema, moist rales) or *peptide sensitivity* (headache, myalgia, fever, nausea, rash, abdominal pain);

— maintain I&O record; check weight daily to maintain proper fluid balance.

3) Comfort and Exercise

The patient will verbalize an understanding of the procedure; the patient will exercise within capabilities and limitations in order to promote weight gain of lean muscle rather than fatty tissue:

— explain rationale for hyperal & give proper explanations for every step of the procedure; answer all the pt.'s questions; allow pt. to verbalize any comments & fears;

— encourage pt. to exercise within his capabilities & restrictions; provide passive ROM exercises PRN (see NCPG #1:47); ambulate when not contraindicated.

Recommended References

Handbook of Total Parenteral Nutrition, by J. Grant. Philadelphia: Saunders, 1980.

"Meeting Patients' Nutritional Needs with Hyperalimentation," by R. Colley and J. Wilson. *Nursing '79,* May:76–83, June:57–61, July:50–53, August:56–63, September 1979:62–69.

"Taking the Worry Out of Hyperal," by C. Giordano et al. *RN,* Part I: June 1981:50–55.

"Range of Motion Exercises." *NCP Guide #1:47,* 2nd Ed., Nurseco, 1980.